# Smoking among healthcare professionals

Derek R. Smith and Peter A. Leggat

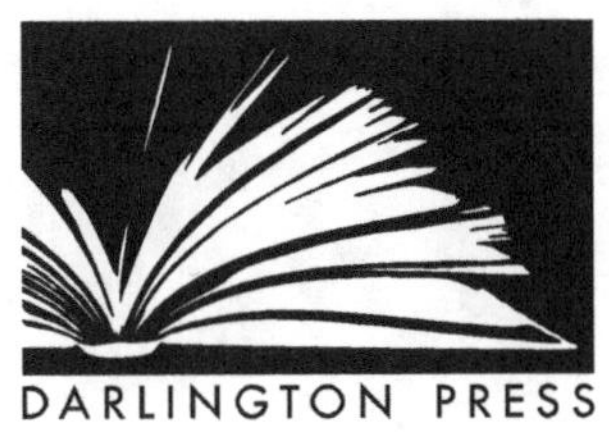

First published 2011 by Darlington Press

Darlington Press is an imprint of SYDNEY UNIVERSITY PRESS



**Reproduction and Communication for other purposes**



Sydney University Press
Fisher Library F03, University of Sydney
NSW 2006 Australia
Email: sup.info@sydney.edu.au

**National Library of Australia Cataloguing-in-Publication entry**

| | |
|---|---|
| Author: | Smith, Derek Richard, 1971- |
| Title: | Smoking among healthcare professionals / Derek R. Smith and Peter A. Leggat. |
| ISBN: | 9781921364174 (pbk.) |
| Notes: | Includes bibliographical references and index. |
| Subjects: | Smoking cessation. |
| | Medical personnel. |
| Other Authors/Contributors: | |
| | Leggat, Peter A. |

Dewey Number: 616.86506

Cover design by Miguel Yamin, the University Publishing Service

# Contents

# List of tables

# Foreword

Smoking can be seen as the unmet challenge confronting all those with responsibilities for personal and public health. The challenge is particularly great as the pleasure of smoking gives instant gratification. Like all deleterious agents whose short-term effects are enjoyed but whose long-term results manifest years after exposure, the long-term debt so accrued seems remote from the moment of the 'here and now'. That debt is always tragic for the individual and places great demands on the society in which smokers live.

Health professionals occupy a pivotal role in the prevention of smoking-induced morbidity and mortality. In the promotion of better health, their position is 'necessary but not sufficient' to reduce individual preventable disease and the epidemic morbidity in societies of both the developed and developing world. However, they cannot do this alone, with support being needed at all levels. In 2011, the Australian federal government approved a milestone legislation mandating the plain packaging of tobacco products. This was one example of collaboration between health professionals and politicians where courage and focused action will undoubtedly help reduce smoking-induced injury and death. It has been shown, for example, that for an investment of less than 200 million dollars, spread over a generation (of 30 years), a return of almost nine billion dollars might be anticipated in healthcare savings.

All competent adults have free choice, a choice that is however, only truly free if its outcomes do not impinge on others. The morbidity and premature mortality that smoking engenders impinges greatly on societal resources – in terms both of monetary demand and the overload of health systems. Thus, the subject addressed in this book is of interest to more than just those who work in the many disciplines of health. It forms an inescapable component of professional life – from that of the paediatrician advising well children and teenagers, to the geriatrician preserving residual intellect in the infirm aged; as well as generalists and specialists of all the health disciplines in between these extremes of life.

The delayed nexus between cause and effect challenges many themes in public health and preventive medicine. The dyads of asbestos-mesothelioma, boxing-dementia and sun exposure–skin cancer affect specific subgroups in the world's population. Smoking, however, transcends the barriers of profession and craft or the latitude of domicile. The already high prevalence of smoking continues to increase in developing nations. Thus, the lessons concerning prevention, already learnt at great individual cost, provide support for those wishing to abstain. Knowledge of smoking-induced cancers, and pulmonary and vascular pathology understood since the 1960s, will continue to have particular relevance to those afflicted by smoking morbidity in future decades.

Inescapably, those who practise in the caring professions serve as role models for the promotion of healthy lifestyles. Such role models are influential in the one-to-one dyad of a doctor, nurse, dentist or therapist and his or her patients. Role models are also influential at a community level. A nurse, surgeon or physiotherapist who continues to smoke, like doctors, dentists and sportspersons, induce perplexity in those who see the juxtaposition of an unhealthy example on one hand and the profession of fitness and health on the other. The ethical impost on all those who care for others is thus significant. In the pages of this book, one sees a snapshot of this subject – the health professional and his or her attitudes to smoking – and a perspective of what is possible in a future, enlightened and healthier world.

*John H. Pearn, AO, RFD*

Professor of Paediatrics and Child Health

Royal Children's Hospital, Brisbane, Australia

# Acknowledgements

The publication of a book, or indeed any endeavour of magnitude, can never be completed alone. As such, I am grateful to various individuals who were instrumental in helping to bring together all of the previously disparate parts. First and foremost, I would like to thank my co-author, Professor Peter A. Leggat from James Cook University, for his generous collaboration and ongoing encouragement in making this book a reality. I would like to thank Glenn Courtenay from the University of Newcastle for his outstanding efforts in updating, editing and proofreading the material. Agata Mrva-Montoya from the Sydney University Press is gratefully acknowledged for her expert assistance in editing and preparing the manuscript. I would also like to thank Fiona Neville and Catherine Doust from the University of Newcastle. As always, I would like to thank my parents Richard and Judy Smith, and my wife, Dr Sarah Tang for instilling within me the importance of lifelong learning and healthy lifestyles. This book is dedicated to my family, for keeping me the healthiest of all.

*Derek R. Smith*


It has been a pleasure working with Professor Derek Smith and other colleagues in collating this research around the topic of smoking among healthcare professionals. Derek, in particular, has been instrumental in driving the completion of this book. While there is some way to go to achieving the enviable goal of zero smoking among healthcare professionals, the discipline of public health has come a long way since the days of Sir Richard Doll in reducing the rates of smoking more broadly in the community. I would like to take the opportunity of thanking my keenest supporters, my wife Associate Professor Ureporn Kedjarune-Leggat and my parents, Bruce and Frances Leggat. I wish to also acknowledge my many mentors in occupational health over the years, including the late Professor Richard Kelman, the late Dr Ralph Shapiro, the late Associate Professor Deane O. Southgate, AM (widely regarded as the founding father of the Australian College of Occupational Medicine), the late Professor Harry Adrounie, Professor Bill Glass and Dr John Heyden.

*Peter A. Leggat*

for Sarah and Pan

# Chapter 1

# Introduction

*This chapter provides some historical background on the issue of smoking, its importance as a worldwide health hazard, as well as the development of smoking attitudes and practices in the general population. Most importantly, this chapter highlights the significance of tobacco control in the healthcare profession, how this group can make a positive difference in the lives of their patients, and why healthcare professionals should not smoke. The first step in meeting this goal is to clearly understand how many of them smoke, in what country, and at what stage in their career. The gathering of such data is the focus of this book.*

## 1.1    Background

Tobacco use represents one of the most important public health issues in the world today. The problem is vast, with over one billion smokers worldwide and many millions more using oral tobacco products.[1] Tobacco kills over five million people every year, accounts for 10% of all adult mortality and is a risk factor for six of the top eight causes of death, worldwide. If current trends continue, tobacco will be responsible for around eight million deaths per year, and up to one billion deaths in the 21st century.[2]

Although humans have a long history of tobacco smoking, the 20th century can be seen as a landmark period during which time considerable changes in tobacco consumption occurred. While humans have used tobacco products in one form or another for thousands of years, it was not until last century that smoking became a common and widespread practice throughout society. National consumption levels subsequently rose, with per capita tobacco consumption in the United States (US) for example, increasing from 6 pounds per person in the 1880s, to approximately 13 pounds per person in the mid 20th century.[3, 4] So well accepted was the practice within the general population that in 1922, at least one commentator had suggested that 'one is more justified in looking with suspicion on the abstainer'.[5] Healthcare professionals were not immune to these social forces, and as a result, a large proportion of them also smoked, with some even advertising cigarettes.[6, 7] The mid 20th century, however, marked the beginning of a decline in cigarette consumption, as the adverse health effects of smoking became increasingly clear and the weight of scientific evidence mounted.

Groundbreaking scientific reports published in the mid to late 1950s[8-10] did much to unsettle public confidence in the safety of tobacco use, and as a result, various advertising campaigns appeared which referred directly to healthcare professionals (usually doctors) in an attempt to assure consumers that tobacco products were safe.[11, 12] Various medical journals began to carry pro-tobacco advertisements during this period,[6] with one article from the late 1950s,[13] for example, suggesting that 'we might as well continue to smoke and enjoy ourselves'. A major blow was struck against tobacco in 1964 with the release of the Surgeon General's Advisory Committee on Smoking and Health landmark report.[14] This document unequivocally concluded that smoking was a health hazard of sufficient importance to warrant remedial action, thereby leading many citizens to question the safety of smoking and to seriously consider quitting. Further evidence was provided by a number of other studies, including a 1965 publication from New York State, where higher death rates were reported in cigarette smokers of the general population when compared to non-smokers.[15] Amidst this growing public concern, tobacco industry strategists determined that healthcare professionals were no longer credible in cigarette advertising, and commercials incorporating them began to slowly disappear.[12] Over time, many healthcare professionals themselves quit smoking and began to take up the fight against tobacco use.

## 1.2    The critical role of healthcare professionals

It is well known that healthcare professionals occupy a vital position in tobacco control and that they can make a real difference in the reduction of community smoking rates.[16] There are a few reasons for this. Firstly, they have regular and close contact with patients, a situation which affords continuous opportunity to not only detect which patients might be smokers and to whom quitting advice may be directed, but also to provide follow-up counselling and support to those who are trying to quit. Secondly, most healthcare professionals are on the frontlines of primary health care, and are well positioned to intervene with patients at various life stages. Thirdly, they are generally well respected by their patients and represent a trusted source of healthcare advice for the public. Indeed, many smokers will inevitably turn to them for advice. Healthcare professionals also represent important role models in the community and serve as exemplars for healthy behaviour,[17] one which includes the public health image they portray outside of the work environment.[18] On the other hand, healthcare professionals who smoke will invariably attract public skepticism,[19] with people inclined to ask why they should stop smoking when their doctor has not. Furthermore, tobacco use by healthcare professionals undermines the important message to smokers that quitting is important.[20] As early as 1976, it had been suggested the healthcare professionals could best persuade patients to quit if they themselves did not smoke.[21] Public expectations of healthcare professionals also began to change. By the 1980s, for example, research from the US had shown that 80% of citizens expected their doctors to be non-smokers.[22]

Despite the weight of scientific evidence and the best efforts of many groups, considerable challenges still remain for tobacco control in health care. The global occupational demographic of healthcare professionals is not an entirely smoke-free one, and as such, it is imperative that measures be taken to address this problem. Given that tobacco control can be a complex process, it is essential that smoking-related interventions be appropriately formulated and targeted to the groups most in need. Much can be learned from an examination of smoking trends within the healthcare sector; the most important being a comprehensive understanding of how many of them smoke, in what country, and at what stage in their career. The gathering of such data is the focus of this book.

## 1.3    Outline of the book

This book comprises six interrelated chapters. Chapter 1 provides some historical background on the issue of smoking, its importance as a worldwide health hazard, as well as the development of smoking attitudes and practices in the general population. It also highlights why tobacco control in the healthcare profession is significant, how this group can make a real difference in the lives of their patients, and most importantly, why healthcare professionals themselves should not smoke. Chapter 2 describes the methodology used for conducting a comprehensive review of all international literature on tobacco smoking among doctors, dentists and nurses in clinical practice and in training. The literature search strategy and target databases are identified, a discussion of the inclusion and exclusion criteria is provided, along with an examination of the main limitations and confounding aspects of the data obtained. Overall, the most important limitation of published data on healthcare workers' smoking habits appears to be the use of inconsistent data collection methodologies, combined with suboptimal coverage and limited response rates when questionnaire surveys were used. One major confounding factor identified across many investigations was a general lack of standardisation regarding the definition of a 'current smoker'.

Chapter 3 describes a comprehensive review of all international literature describing the prevalence of tobacco smoking among doctors, dentists and nurses. Two distinct trends were evident across all three professional groups. Firstly, most developed countries have shown a steady decline in smoking rates in the health profession during recent years. Secondly, however, this trend does not appear to be internationally uniform, with some developed countries and newly developing regions reporting high tobacco usage rates in the health care sector. Comparison between the health professions suggests that dentists are generally the least likely to be current tobacco users, followed by doctors and then nurses. Overall, this chapter suggests that while healthcare professionals' smoking habits vary from region to region, they are not uniformly low when viewed from an international perspective. It is important that smoking within this group continues to decline in future years, so that healthcare professionals can remain at the forefront of anti-smoking programs and lead the way as public health exemplars in the 21st century.

Chapter 4 provides a comprehensive review of all international literature describing the prevalence of tobacco smoking among the students of medicine, dentistry and nursing. Research publications tend to suggest that the prevalence of smoking among medical students varies widely between students of different countries, and also between male and female students within the same countries. Consistently low smoking rates were documented in regions such as Australia and the US, while generally high rates were seen in countries such as Greece, Italy, Spain and Turkey. While many cross-sectional investigations suggested that the prevalence of smoking seems to increase during the more senior grades, it is difficult to assess whether this trend directly reflects university seniority, increasing age or both.

Chapter 5 describes the decline of smoking among Australian and American doctors in the mid to late 20th century. Published literature suggests that although around one-quarter of Australian doctors were smoking by the 1950s, this rate declined over time to a level below that of the general population. Similarly, in the US, many doctors had begun questioning the safety of tobacco products, a situation which resulted in a continuous decline in use. By the late 20th century, few Australian or American doctors were current smokers, and many of their younger demographic had probably never smoked at all. Overall, this chapter suggests not only that very few Australian and American doctors smoke when compared internationally, but that an active professional community can make a real difference to the lifestyle choices of its own members. Much can be learned from this pivotal era of public health, where the importance of scientific knowledge, professional leadership and social responsibility helped set positive examples in the fight against tobacco use.

Chapter 6 provides a concluding discussion on the topic of smoking among healthcare professionals. Overall, it is clear that much can be learned from an examination of smoking trends within the healthcare workforce, and indeed, this extends to the next generation – the healthcare students of today. While there are no-doubt common issues faced by healthcare workforces around the world, significant cultural and social influences are also prevalent, making it difficult to adopt a 'one-size-fits-all' solution. Tobacco control among the healthcare professionals of today, and those of tomorrow, will clearly need to adopt a multifaceted approach in tackling the unacceptably high prevalence of smoking that is still being reported in some countries.

# Chapter 2

# Methodology

*This chapter describes the methodology used when examining the international literature on tobacco smoking among healthcare professionals. The search strategy and target databases are described, along with a discussion of the inclusion and exclusion criteria, as well as some limitations identified in the published literature. One of the most important limitations appears to be the use of inconsistent data collection methodologies among the published studies of tobacco smoking among healthcare professionals, as well as suboptimal response rates when questionnaire surveys were utilised as the primary methodology. One further limitation identified across many investigations was the general lack of a standard definition of a 'current smoker'.*

## 2.1    Search strategy and databases

To enable a comprehensive understanding of the international literature on tobacco use in the healthcare profession, an extensive literature search was undertaken which targeted all published research in the field of tobacco smoking among healthcare professionals and students. The search covered a total of six different elements, each corresponding to the specific group of healthcare professionals or students under study; that being, doctors, dentists, nurses, medical students, dental students and nursing students. A preliminary search of the US National Library of Medicine's (NLM) *PubMed / Medline* database was conducted using relevant *Medical Subject Headings* (MeSH) and associated keyword variations. As English has become the international language of scientific research and basically all literature search engines now include it, our search strategy originally focused on manuscripts written in this language. As the review progressed, some additional articles written in other languages were included if they contained English language abstracts.

Literature searches were conducted using logical keyword variations such as 'smoke', 'smoking' and 'tobacco', as well as some broader terms such as 'substance use' and 'substance abuse'. To limit results to the target population of healthcare professionals, searches were refined using the Boolean command 'AND', combined with the basic words 'doctor', 'dentist' and 'nurse'. The Boolean operator * was also included to detect variations of the same word, such as 'doctors', 'dentists' and 'nurses'. The search was then expanded using specific alternative keywords with the same meaning such as 'physician', 'medical practitioner', 'dental profession', 'nursing profession'; as well as broader terms such as 'healthcare professional', 'healthcare worker', and so on. Although a large number of smoking-related studies were identified using these methods, results were not evenly distributed across all six groups. By far the greatest proportion of published research identified during our literature searches for this book appears to have focused on doctors and dentists.

While our initial strategy was effective at locating smoking-related research conducted among doctors and dentists, it did result in a lower than expected number of studies from the nursing profession. Such a result was not entirely unexpected however, as it has been previously noted that only a small proportion of nursing periodicals are included in medical databases. Indeed, in 2005, it was estimated that less than 1% of the nursing journals were actually listed in the Thomson Reuters *Journal Citation Reports*® (JCR).[1] Any literature review which locates its material through medical search engines alone therefore, could be expected to miss some important articles. As such, our literature search for nursing professionals and nursing students also included an investigation of the *Cumulative Index to Nursing and Allied Health Literature* (CINAHL) and the *British Nursing Index* (BNI). Proportionally fewer studies we identified in the initial searches had been conducted in developing countries, although this was not entirely unexpected given that biomedical research tends to have a general bias against countries with lower economic rankings.[2] For these reasons, it was also considered necessary to thoroughly examine the reference lists of all manuscripts identified using the initial search protocol, in order to locate as many additional publications as possible. This strategy proved particularly useful for locating publications relevant to the topic under study, but which had been published in journals not included in the databases initially targeted. Indeed, a large proportion of all manuscripts were eventually located using this latter method.

## 2.2    Preparation of data

A copy of each published manuscript was obtained and examined. Manuscript details were then entered into a spreadsheet program, arranged alphabetically by country and sorted in descending order by year of publication. From this process, six tables were created, one for each of the six groups of healthcare professionals and students examined in the book. Each table included information on the country where the study was conducted, the overall smoking rate, the sample size obtained in the study, its response rate, and finally, the study authors and the year of publication. Smoking rates were listed as the prevalence of smoking among the entire group, and also as smoking rates for males and females. For consistency, all smoking rates and response rates were rounded to the nearest whole number. As some studies had investigated multiple occupational groups which included healthcare professionals (as opposed to studies which had investigated the smoking rates of healthcare professionals exclusively), some response rates were indicative of the entire group response. This book utilises the Vancouver Referencing System as specified by the International Committee of Medical Journal Editors (ICMJE) *Uniform Requirements for Manuscripts Submitted to Biomedical Journals*.[3] As the results of some investigations of smoking among healthcare professionals were published over more than one journal article, some studies have two or three corresponding references.

## 2.3 Limitations and confounding factors

The literature search undertaken for this book revealed a few, relatively common limitations in the published literature on smoking among healthcare professionals. Firstly, there is the issue of research methodology, as the most frequently used protocol for determining an individual's smoking status appears to be the self-reporting questionnaire. This is probably because questionnaire surveys represent a cost-effective and convenient methodology for researching large and dispersed occupational groups, such as healthcare professionals. While biochemical measures are being increasingly used to investigate smoking habits, the validity and accuracy of self-reported smoking surveys have been demonstrated in a variety of studies,[4, 5] making it a viable option which many researchers had ultimately chosen. Another potential limitation of the published literature appears to be a general lack of standardisation regarding the definition of a 'current smoker' – an issue that was apparent across research studies from all six groups. Although most authors referred to their subjects as being either 'current smokers' or 'non-smokers', some used various recall periods ranging from one week to one month in their definition of the term 'current', while some studies did not list a recall period at all. This may have arisen due to the inherent difficulties in assessing smoking habits over time, and the fact that most investigations simply described the prevalence of tobacco smoking among the surveyed group at a particular point in time when the survey was undertaken. In many cases, this simply involved asking the subjects, 'are you a smoker?'

In studies where there was ambiguity regarding smoking definition, composition of the sample or research design, the corresponding author of the selected manuscript was contacted, where possible. Not all authors could be contacted, and of those who were, not all responded. No corresponding authors were contacted prior to the literature search, nor were any encouraged to submit their own work for inclusion in the book, prior to being contacted. Finally, with regard to potential limitations in the published literature, there was the issue of what the subjects were actually smoking. While for the most part, a 'smoker' was defined in most studies as one who smoked cigarettes, not all healthcare professionals were defined as smoking cigarettes exclusively, an issue which appeared to be most common in the research conducted among doctors. A study of Hispanic doctors in the US,[6] for example, found that 7% of their subjects smoked cigars, and none smoked cigarettes. Similarly, two UK[7, 8] studies revealed that a large proportion of doctors only smoked pipes or cigars, rather than cigarettes.

# Chapter 3

# Tobacco use among healthcare professionals

*This chapter provides a review of international literature describing the prevalence of smoking among doctors, dentists and nurses. Results suggest that many countries have experienced a steady decline in smoking rates in the health profession during recent years. This finding does not appear to be internationally uniform, however, with some regions still reporting high smoking rates in the healthcare sector. Comparison between the health professions indicates that dentists are the least likely to be smokers, followed by doctors and then nurses.*

## 3.1    Smoking rates among doctors

More than 100 published studies on doctors' smoking habits were located and examined for this section of the chapter, as shown in Table 3.1. Response rates of the published studies ranged from 2%[1] to 100%,[2, 3] with most being above 60%. Only seven investigations had response rates below 50%, and six did not list their response rate. Sample sizes ranged from 45[4] to 10,807[5] with the largest sample sizes coming from the *Doctor's Health Study* in the United Kingdom (UK),[5] the *Physicians Health Study* in the US[6–8] and also from New Zealand census data.[9–11] New Zealand is one of the few countries in the world that includes tobacco smoking questions on their census form.[11]

When viewed from an international perspective, the overall rate of smoking among doctors in most developed countries appears to have steadily declined over the past 30 years. In the US, for example, many recent studies have consistently shown the prevalence of smoking among doctors to be lower than 10%. Three investigations of their Australian counterparts in the 1990s[12–14] revealed a smoking rate of around 5%, while in New Zealand, analysis of census data has also suggested a similar rate during this period,[11] with more recent data further supporting the evidence of a downward trend.[15, 16] Smoking has been well studied longitudinally among doctors in the UK,[5, 17, 18] although a certain proportion continue to smoke pipes and cigars, rather than cigarettes. Nevertheless, overall tobacco consumption has still declined markedly, with the proportion of British doctors who smoked cigars, pipes or cigarettes falling from 62% to 18% between 1951 and 1990.[5] Not all regions of the world have demonstrated a clear decline in tobacco usage among doctors, however. Multiple investigations conducted over the past 20 years in France,[19–21] Italy[22–26] and Japan,[27–36] for example, have consistently documented smoking rates in excess of 20% in this group. A relatively high prevalence of smoking is also evident among doctors in some developing countries (Bosnia & Herzegovina,[37] Estonia,[38, 39] Turkey[40] and Vietnam[41]), but not all (Nigeria[42] and Brazil[43]).

The lowest overall smoking rates have been consistently documented in the US (2%),[44-46] with similar low rates recorded in Australia (3%)[14] and the UK (3%).[47] The highest smoking rate was recorded in Greece,[48] where roughly half of all doctors (49%) reported to be smokers. Almost half of all Chinese (45%)[49] and Japanese doctors (42%)[28] were reported to be smokers. Similar results were also documented in Kuwait (38%) and the United Arab Emirates (36%),[50] particularly among males (of whom 45% and 44% smoked, respectively). In some studies, almost half of all male Indian (48%)[51] and Sudanese (46%)[52] doctors were reported to be smokers.

Smoking rates have been shown to vary by gender, with the rates among male doctors being documented in Japan (68%)[53] and in China (61%).[49] High smoking rates among female doctors have been demonstrated in Greece,[54] as well as in some investigations from Italy[26] and France.[19, 20] Conversely, other research on doctors' smoking habits from China,[55] Hong Kong,[56] Malaysia[3] and the UK (Wales)[57] has revealed no female smokers at all. This may suggest a cultural reluctance for professional women to smoke in certain regions. Although a relatively large number of studies reported that male doctors smoked at higher rates than their female counterparts, this finding was not without exception. An Italian study,[26] for example, found that more female doctors smoked when compared to their male counterparts, while in Australia,[13] Israel,[58] New Zealand[11, 15, 16] and the US,[59] smoking prevalence was almost the same between the genders. A large proportion of manuscripts did not divide their smoking rates by gender, however, making it impossible to do further gender comparisons. Age may also be a factor as some studies have documented age-related differences in doctors' smoking rates, with older doctors for the most part, more likely to be smokers. Nevertheless, in China,[55] Japan,[28, 32] Mexico[60] and India,[51] tobacco usage was actually more prevalent in younger doctors.

Some studies have simultaneously investigated the tobacco usage habits of dentists, nurses and other hospital staff while surveying doctors. Two investigations from the US[61, 62] found that fewer doctors smoked when compared to dentists, while another study demonstrated very similar, albeit very low, smoking rates among both doctors and dentists.[45] In 1979, a study of smoking among doctors and lawyers found that doctors were less likely to be smokers than were lawyers.[63] Most studies found that fewer doctors smoked when compared to nurses at the same facility, although an investigation from Finland[64] suggested the opposite situation may sometimes occur. This is not entirely surprising, as research suggests that doctors tend to give up smoking before other occupational groups and the general public.[65] There are a few reasons for this. Firstly, they may recognise the negative medical consequences more quickly than the general public. In this regard, doctors are well equipped to evaluate scientific knowledge, and can reasonably be expected to act upon new discoveries, if warranted.[66] Secondly, their devotion to health naturally conflicts with unhealthy behaviours. Thirdly, tobacco smoking usually incurs a negative image in the healthcare profession long before it does so in the wider community.[65] Furthermore, smoking rates in some developed countries tend to decrease over time due to a generational effect and changing social norms with more people giving up smoking, including doctors.[67]

Tobacco smoking by medical specialty also revealed some interesting, though inconsistent results. One study, for example, found that doctors specialising in family medicine were less likely to be smokers than doctors generally,[7] while two other studies suggested that more general practitioners smoked when compared to medical specialists.[67, 68] In a study from the Netherlands, more consultants smoked than house officers.[13, 69] Trainee psychiatrists[13] and psychiatry residents[70] were the most likely to smoke in some investigations, while in some other studies, the highest rates were demonstrated among surgeons[48] or obstetricians.[9] Japanese chest physicians have been shown to have a lower smoking rate than Japanese doctors in other specialities.[29-31] Exactly how much a doctor's medical specialty influences their smoking habits is uncertain, however. A study of Malaysian doctors, for example,[3] found that around half were already smoking before they entered medical school. Based on the findings of multiple investigations therefore, it is very difficult to ascertain which medical specialty has the highest or lowest smoking rate.

Regarding anti-smoking practices, most doctors in a UK study[71] felt they should advise patients to quit, and in France,[21] over half of the tobacco-using doctors had made at least one serious attempt to quit smoking themselves. In Italy,[77] however, more than half the doctors who smoked had made no attempt to quit smoking, and in Japan,[36] only 60% of doctors who smoked stated any intention of reducing their tobacco consumption or quitting altogether. Other authors have already suggested that Japanese doctors may not be setting a good example in this regard.[72] The institutions where doctors work may also play an important role in tobacco control, with a US study[73] demonstrating that a hospital no-smoking policy was useful in helping to reduce the overall smoking rate among staff. US hospitals were probably the first group to declare a national smoking ban and were also significant in their influence on social norms and the ultimate reduction of overall smoking rates.[74] Even so, the location of the actual hospital in which doctors work may not always affect the smoking rates. One Italian study, for example, found different smoking rates by region,[25] although in Nigeria,[42] the smoking rates of doctors in two different hospitals were exactly the same. A doctor's smoking habit may also be reflective of their spouse and vice versa, with two studies from the UK (Scotland)[75] and New Zealand[76] revealing that around half of all male doctors who smoked, also had wives who smoked.

The extent to which the professional practice of doctors is affected by their smoking habits has been examined in certain investigations. One of the most marked differences in this regard was found in Greece,[48] where only half the doctors who smoked were involved in smoking cessation counselling, compared to 100% of their non-smoking colleagues. Several Japanese studies also revealed differences in smoking-cessation advice[36] and discussion of a patient's smoking history,[35] with both being significantly more commonplace among non-smoking doctors. Similar findings were also seen in Finland.[77] Furthermore, a study of Estonian doctors who smoked found that they were reluctant to impose on patients' privacy by asking about their tobacco usage habits.[39] Knowledge of smoking-related damage has also revealed correlations with smoking behaviour in a study of Italian doctors,[24] although the analysis was performed on a multidisciplinary group of health professionals, rather than doctors alone. Nonetheless, not all research findings have been consistent in this regard. In a study from Israel, for example, doctors were asked whether during consultations, they advised patients to stop smoking. Interestingly, no difference was found between doctors who smoked and those who did not.[58]

Nevertheless, health counselling behaviours are not necessarily fixed, and may change over time. A longitudinal study of Chinese doctors for example, revealed that the effects of smoking on counselling behaviour varied between 1987 and 1996.[49] In 1987, for example, smoking behaviour was found to be an influential factor, whereas by 1996, it had ceased to be so. Other confounding issues were also raised by the aforementioned Chinese study. Firstly, only one-third of doctors believed that they were the most influential person who could help patients quit. On the other hand, over three-quarters believed that doctors can set a good example for patients by not smoking. Most disturbing, however, was the finding that anti-smoking counselling practices appear to be diminishing among Chinese doctors in recent years.[49] These discrepancies between countries suggest that not only are doctor-targeted smoking interventions urgently needed in public health, but that they should also be culturally specific.

Table 3.1    Smoking rates among doctors

| Country | Smoking rate [a] | | | Study details | | |
| | All | Male | Female | Sample size | Response rate [b] | Authors |
| --- | --- | --- | --- | --- | --- | --- |
| Australia | 14% | 14% | 17% | 1276 | 69% | Rankin et al., 1975[78] |
| Australia | 21% | 22% | 16% | 275 | 80% | Dodds et al.,1979[79] |
| Australia | 6% | 6% | 5% | 1361 | 55% | Roche et al., 1995[13] |
| Australia | 4% | – | – | 908 | 55% | Roche et al., 1996[12] |
| Australia | 3% | 4% | 2% | 855 | 67% | Young & Ward, 1997[14] |
| Belgium | 32% | 34% | 16% | 2157 | 67% | Joossens et al., 1987[80] |
| Bosnia & Herzegovina | 40% | – | – | 112 | 73% | Hodgetts et al., 2004[37] |
| Brazil | 6% | 9% | 5% | 830 | 12% | de Assis Viegas et al., 2007[43] |

| | Smoking rate [a] | | | Study details | | |
|---|---|---|---|---|---|---|
| Country | All | Male | Female | Sample size | Response rate [b] | Authors |
| Canada | 19% | – | – | 88 | 52% | Senior, 1982[81] |
| Canada | – | 13% | 7% | 1540 | 51% | De Koninck et al., 1995[82] |
| China | 45% | 61% | 12% | 493 | 82% | Li et al., 1999[49] |
| China | 16% | 32% | 0% | 286 | 79% | Smith et al., 2006[55] |
| China | 23% | 41% | 1% | 3552 | 100% | Jiang et al., 2007[2] |
| China | 36% | – | – | 358 | 70% | Yan et al., 2008[83] |
| China | 26% | 35% | 3% | 673 | 85% | Zhou et al., 2010[84] |
| Costa Rica | 19% | – | – | 217 | 76% | Grossman et al., 1999[85] |
| Denmark | 25% | – | – | 445 | 91% | Willaing et al., 2003[86] |
| Denmark | 15% | – | – | 729 | 75% | Kannegaard et al., 2005[87] |
| Estonia | – | 25% | 11% | 2668 | 68% | Parna et al., 2005[38, 39] |
| Finland | – | 10% | 6% | 1231 | 76% | Jormanainen et al., 1997[68] |
| Finland | 10% | – | – | 725 | 72% | Heloma et al., 1998[64] |
| Finland | – | 7% | 3% | 1221 | 76% | Barengo et al., 2004[88] |
| Finland | – | 5% | 3% | 3057 | 69% | Barengo et al., 2005[77] |
| France | 21% | 22% | 14% | 4318 | 37% | Tessier et al., 1993[21] |
| France | 34% | 36% | 25% | 1013 | 65% | Josseran et al., 2000[20] |
| France | 32% | 34% | 25% | 2073 | 67% | Josseran et al., 2005[19] |

Smoking among healthcare professionals

| Country | Smoking rate [a] | | | Study details | | |
| --- | --- | --- | --- | --- | --- | --- |
| | All | Male | Female | Sample size | Response rate [b] | Authors |
| Greece | 49% | – | – | 148 | – | Polyzos *et al.*, 1995[48] |
| Greece | 39% | 40% | 37% | 1284 | – | Sotiropoulos *et al.*, 2007[54] |
| Hong Kong | 5% | 7% | 0% | 133 | 88% | Cheng & Lam, 1990[56] |
| India | 32% | 48% | 3% | 218 | 99% | Sarkar *et al.*, 1990[51] |
| India | – | 11% | – | 229 | 86% | Mohan *et al.*, 2006[90] |
| Iran | 9% | – | – | 111 | – | Ahmadi *et al.*, 2001[91] |
| Ireland | 16% | – | – | 171 | 85% | Power *et al.*, 2004[92] |
| Israel | 16% | 16% | 15% | 260 | 87% | Samuels, 1997[58] |
| Italy | 31% | – | – | 709 | 86% | Franceschi *et al.*, 1986[93] |
| Italy | 39% | – | – | 959 | 57% | Nardini *et al.*, 1998[24] |
| Italy | 25% | – | – | 605 | 62% | Nardini *et al.*, 1998[23] |
| Italy | 31% | 29% | 34% | 2453 | 68% | Zanetti *et al.*, 1998[26] |
| Italy | 24% | 25% | 23% | 501 | – | La Vecchia *et al.*, 2000[22] |
| Italy | 28% | 32% | 20% | 526 | 72% | Pizzo *et al.*, 2003[25] |
| Italy | 34% | – | – | 165 | – | Ficarra *et al.*, 2010[94] |
| Japan | – | 68% | – | 6815 | 51% | Kono *et al.*, 1985[53] |
| Japan | 25% | 26% | 6% | 3640 | 59% | Kawane, 1991, 1993, 2001[29-31] |
| Japan | 29% | – | – | 163 | 60% | Kawane & Soejima, 1996[32] |

| | Smoking rate [a] | | | Study details | | |
| Country | All | Male | Female | Sample size | Response rate [b] | Authors |
| --- | --- | --- | --- | --- | --- | --- |
| Japan | 21% | 24% | 7% | 323 | 71% | Kawakami *et al.*, 1997[36] |
| Japan | 26% | 28% | 5% | 709 | 91% | Kawahara *et al.*, 2000[35] |
| Japan | 42% | 43% | 9% | 4190 | 84% | Kaetsu *et al.*, 2002[28] |
| Japan | 32% | 33% | 5% | 3565 | 63% | Kaetsu *et al.*, 2002[27] |
| Japan | – | 27% | 7% | 3771 | 84% | Ohida *et al.*, 2001[33] |
| Japan | 16% | 22% | 5% | 3633 | 81% | Kaneita *et al.*, 2008[34]; Kaneita *et al.*, 2010[95] |
| Japan | – | 15% | 5% | 3486 | 77% | Kaneita *et al.*, 2010[95] |
| Kuwait | 38% | 45% | 16% | 252 | 84% | Bener *et al.*, 1993[50] |
| Malaysia | 18% | 25% | 0% | 120 | 100% | Yaacob & Abdullah, 1993[3] |
| Mexico | 27% | 30% | 21% | 3488 | 98% | Tapia-Conyer *et al.*, 1997[60] |
| Netherlands | 32% | 37% | 14% | 362 | 63% | Waalkens *et al.*, 1992[69] |
| Netherlands | 38% | 41% | 24% | 263 | 82% | Dekker *et al.*, 1993[67] |
| Netherlands | 7% | – | – | 1180 | 40% | Kotz *et al.*, 2006[89] |
| New Zealand | – | 20% | 17% | 4089 | 97% | Hay, 1980[9] |
| New Zealand | 15% | 15% | 13% | 4937 | 97% | Hay, 1984[10] |
| New Zealand | 5% | 5% | 5% | 7335 | 97% | Hay, 1998[11] |

| | Smoking rate [a] | | | Study details | | |
|---|---|---|---|---|---|---|
| Country | All | Male | Female | Sample size | Response rate [b] | Authors |
| New Zealand | – | 4% | 3% | 10,509 | 97% | Edwards *et al.*, 2008; Ponniah & Bloomfield, 2008[15, 16] |
| Nigeria | 3% | – | – | 373 | 60% | Nollen *et al.*, 2004[42] |
| Norway | – | 35% | 22% | 1138 | 95% | Aaro *et al.*, 1977[96] |
| Saudi Arabia | 34% | – | – | 716 | 81% | Saeed, 1991[97] |
| Sudan | – | 46% | 1% | 753 | 72% | Ballal, 1984[52] |
| Switzerland | 12% | 13% | 11% | 1784 | 65% | Sebo *et al.*, 2007[98] |
| Switzerland | 17% | – | – | 1856 | 55% | Sadowski *et al.*, 2009[99] |
| Turkey | 38% | – | – | 153 | – | Akvardar *et al.*, 2004[100] |
| Turkey | 38% | – | – | 257 | 85% | Gunes *et al.*, 2005[40] |
| Turkey | 16% | – | – | 374 | 2% | Uysal *et al.*, 2007[1] |
| United Arab Emirates | 36% | 44% | 8% | 275 | 92% | Bener *et al.*, 1993[50] |
| United Kingdom | 19% | – | – | 607 | 81% | Seiler, 1983[75] |
| United Kingdom | 3% | – | – | 94 | 72% | Davies & Rajan, 1989[47] |
| United Kingdom | 4% | – | – | 2176 | 75% | Fowler *et al.*, 1989[101] |
| United Kingdom | 14% | 17% | 0% | 310 | 60% | Nutbeam & Catford, 1990[57] |
| United Kingdom | 5% | – | – | 1069 | 82% | Hussain *et al.*, 1993[102] |
| United Kingdom | – | 18% | – | 10,807 | 94% | Doll *et al.*, 1994[5] |

| | Smoking rate [a] | | | Study details | | |
|---|---|---|---|---|---|---|
| Country | All | Male | Female | Sample size | Response rate [b] | Authors |
| United Kingdom | 4% | – | – | 303 | 75% | McEwen & West, 2001[71] |
| United States | 14% | – | – | 289 | 70% | Wyshak et al., 1980[63] |
| United States | 12% | – | – | 594 | 27% | Sachs, 1983, 1984[103, 104] |
| United States | – | 15% | – | 151 | 76% | Wells et al., 1984[105] |
| United States | 8% | – | – | 221 | 62% | Fortmann et al., 1985[106] |
| United States | 4% | – | – | 211 | 67% | Linn et al., 1986[107] |
| United States | 6% | – | – | 6050 | 69% | Stillman et al., 1990[73] |
| United States | 4% | – | – | 1754 | 60% | Hughes et al., 1992[70] |
| United States | 5% | 5% | 4% | 2341 | 86% | Scott et al., 1992[59] |
| United States | 6% | – | – | 5426 | 59% | Hughes et al., 1992[108] |
| United States | 9% | 10% | 2% | 393 | 83% | Hensrud & Sprafka, 1993[109] |
| United States | 2% | – | – | 132 | 77% | Brink et al., 1994[45] |
| United States | – | – | 4% | 4501 | 59% | Frank 1995; Frank & Lutz 1999; Frank et al., 2000[6-8] |
| United States | 4% | – | – | 121 | 32% | Hill & Braithwaite, 1997[61] |
| United States | 11% | – | – | 150 | 65% | Hepburn et al., 2000[110] |
| United States | 2% | – | – | 750 | 61% | An et al., 2004[44] |

| | Smoking rate [a] | | | Study details | | |
|---|---|---|---|---|---|---|
| Country | All | Male | Female | Sample size | Response rate [b] | Authors |
| United States | 3% | – | – | 254 | 37% | Misra & Vadaparampil, 2004[111] |
| United States | 4% | – | – | 104 | 63% | Kenna & Wood, 2005[62] |
| United States | 7% | – | – | 45 | 56% | Soto Mas *et al.*, 2005[4] |
| United States | 2% | – | – | 437 | 50% | Tong *et al.*, 2010[46] |
| Vietnam | 23% | – | – | 730 | 86% | An *et al.*, 2008[41] |

[a] Smoking rates rounded to the nearest whole number, [b] Response rates rounded to the nearest whole number

## 3.2 Smoking rates among dentists

More than 40 published studies were located and examined for this section of the chapter, as shown in Table 3.2. Most authors targeted dentists within a single country, although Allard[112] surveyed dentists from a number of regions as part of the European Union (EU) Working Group on Tobacco and Oral Health. Sample sizes varied greatly, ranging from 33 to 2628,[61, 113] with response rates of between 8%[114] and 100%.[115] Some studies obtained fairly large sample sizes and high response rates, for example in Sweden, where 2500 dentists were surveyed and 90% responded.[113] On the other hand, an investigation of almost 5000 oral and maxillofacial surgeons in the US resulted in a fairly low response rate of 28%.[116] One Australian study appeared to have a 100% response rate,[117] although according to the authors, non-respondents to the initial survey approach were replaced until a sufficient number of participants could be obtained.

When investigated from an international perspective, the overall prevalence of smoking appears to be relatively low among dentists. There were some notable exceptions, namely Brazil,[115] Italy[118] and Jordan,[119] where around one-third of dentists were tobacco users; and in Jordan, where one-fifth of dentists were smoking 20 or more cigarettes per day.[119] Despite these findings, smoking prevalence appears to be steadily declining among dentists in recent years, with over 10 studies reporting smoking rates below 10%.

The lowest smoking rate among dentists has been documented in the US (1%),[45] with similar low rates also recorded in Thailand (2%),[120] Australia (3%),[121] Finland (3%),[112] New Zealand (3%)[122] and Canada (4%).[123] On the other hand, relatively high smoking rates have been reported among Japanese (29%),[124] Iranian (24%),[125] New Zealand and Vietnamese dentists (both 11%),[41, 126] and among dentists in European countries such as Sweden (10% to 13%),[112, 113] the Netherlands (12% to 16%),[112, 127] Ireland (15%),[128] Denmark (12%)[112] and Spain (10%).[129]

Aside from the overall prevalence of smoking in the dental profession, additional information has also been documented regarding tobacco usage patterns. Some studies, for example, have distinguished between dentists who were ex-smokers and dentists who had never smoked. In this regard, the prevalence of former smokers ranged from 11%[130] to 48%,[116] with many between 20% and 45%.[112, 118, 121, 123, 128, 131-133] The proportion of dentists who had never smoked was similarly encouraging, with rates of between 55%[134] and 82%.[135] A large number of studies reported that male dentists smoked at higher rates than their female counterparts. This finding was not without exception, however. In Ireland, for example, the prevalence of smoking among male and female dentists was exactly the same (15%).[128] Furthermore, in Spain, the reported smoking rate of male dentists (10%) was only slightly higher than that of their female counterparts (9%).[129] A large proportion of studies did not report their smoking rates by sex, making it impossible to do further gender comparisons. Age was another interesting correlate regarding tobacco use, with higher smoking rates reported among older dentists in some studies.[116, 118, 130]

Length of time spent in the dental profession was an additional correlate demonstrated by some authors,[130, 134] although again, this probably reflects older age of the dentists studied more than anything else. A greater awareness of the negative health effects of tobacco use among younger dentists may, on the other hand, contribute to their comparatively lower smoking rates. This relates not only to decreased smoking initiation among younger dentists, but also the decision to quit smoking among their older peers, who may be more nicotine dependent and perhaps, less likely to give up. Decreasing smoking rates among dentists may also reflect changes in the society at large, with more people giving up smoking, generally. As a pseudo-marker of age (particularly where age of the participants was not directly stated), year of graduation was also shown to affect smoking rates during some investigations of dentists.[114, 117, 123, 132, 133]

Very few studies of dentists appear to have made a distinction between light or heavy smokers. Aside from a Jordanian study,[119] only two investigations have clearly described the degree of smoking, both of which found the majority of tobacco users were not heavy smokers.[136, 137] Similarly, many investigators did not specifically investigate the type of tobacco consumed by the dentist. Although cigarette usage was common,[62, 136, 138-140] the use of pipes and cigars,[79, 114, 119, 126, 141] snuff[113, 116] or water pipes[119] was also reported in some studies. Some studies examined multiple groups of healthcare professionals at the same time as dentists. When compared to other members of the dental profession for example, research suggests that fewer dentists smoke than dental hygienists.[135, 138] When compared to doctors who were also surveyed at the same time however, results were mixed. Some research suggests that dentists may smoke at higher rates than doctors,[61, 62] while others found their rate to be lower.[45]

There are certain demographic and professional similarities between dentists and doctors, with doctors in most developed societies tending to give up smoking sooner than the general population.[65] Given their undoubted similarities with doctors, it is reasonable to assume that dentists may also be influenced in a similar manner.

Although dental professionals have many opportunities to reduce the prevalence of smoking,[142] dentistry may have not yet maximised its efforts in combating the tobacco epidemic.[143,144] Dentists do not routinely incorporate tobacco cessation into their practice.[142] Dentists clearly need to be involved in the prevention and management of oral diseases, while striving to manage the overall health of patients.[145] Dentists also need to expand the bounds of dental practice and embrace smoking-cessation activities as part of comprehensive oral care for patients. Indeed, it has been suggested that such professional behaviour should no longer be a matter of choice.[146] The fact that any dentists continue to smoke is surprising, as dentistry has become increasingly aware of the damaging effect tobacco consumption has on the oral cavity,[147] as well as many other aspects of general health. Dentists incur a certain responsibility as exemplars for patients with regard to healthy behaviour, and a dentist who is a smoker may be less likely to counsel a patient who smokes. In Norway, for example, it was shown that non-smoking dentists reported higher tobacco-cessation intervention levels than their colleagues who smoked.[135] Various barriers that may impede tobacco-cessation activities in the dental office have been suggested in this regard.[142]

Table 3.2        Smoking rates among dentists

| | Smoking rate [a] | | | Study details | | |
|---|---|---|---|---|---|---|
| Country | All | Male | Female | Sample size | Response rate [b] | Authors |
| Australia | 23% | 24% | 8% | 305 | 87% | Dodds *et al.*, 1979[148] |
| Australia | 6% | – | – | 128 | – | Mullins, 1994[117] |
| Australia | 3% | – | – | 95 | 70% | Clover *et al.*, 1999[121] |
| Australia | 4% | – | – | 250 | 57% | Trotter & Worcester, 2003[149] |
| Australia | 4% | 5% | <1% | 281 | 72% | Smith & Leggat, 2005[130] |
| Brazil | 37% | 42% | 31% | 446 | 100% | Rodrigues *et al.*, 2008[115] |
| Canada | 4% | – | – | 765 | 64% | Campbell & Macdonald, 1994[123] |
| Denmark | 12% | – | – | 414 | 52% | Allard, 2000[112] |

| | Smoking rate [a] | | | Study details | | |
|---|---|---|---|---|---|---|
| Country | All | Male | Female | Sample size | Response rate [b] | Authors |
| Finland | 11% | 11% | 2% | 435 | 81% | Telivuo et al., 1991[141] |
| Finland | 3% | – | – | 412 | 53% | Allard, 2000[112] |
| Iran | 24% | 30% | 12% | 1033 | – | Ghasemi et al., 2007[125] |
| Ireland | 15% | 15% | 15% | 427 | 43% | McCartan et al., 1993[128] |
| Italy | 33% | 35% | 21% | 217 | 87% | Lodi et al., 1997[118] |
| Japan | 29% | – | – | 1133 | 37% | Nishio et al., 2009[124] |
| Jordan | 35% | 43% | 15% | 613 | 72% | Burgan, 2003[119] |
| Netherlands | 12% | – | – | 632 | 74% | Allard, 2000[112] |
| Netherlands | 16% | – | – | 709 | 75% | Gorter et al., 2000[127] |
| New Zealand | 11% | – | – | 349 | 88% | Skegg et al., 1995[126] |
| New Zealand | 3% | – | – | 566 | 77% | Ayers et al., 2009[122] |
| Norway | 7% | – | – | 982 | 68% | Lund et al., 2004[135] |
| Spain | 10% | 10% | 9% | 538 | 14% | Peidró et al., 2008[129] |
| Sweden | 13% | 15% | 11% | 2628 | 90% | Halling et al., 1995[113] |
| Sweden | 10% | – | – | 520 | 65% | Allard, 2000[112] |
| Thailand | 2% | – | – | 178 | 81% | Leggat et al., 2001[120] |
| United Kingdom | 6% | – | – | 448 | 76% | Chestnutt & Binnie, 1995[150] |
| United Kingdom | 9% | – | – | 674 | 78% | John et al., 1997[133] |
| United Kingdom | 12% | – | – | 427 | 72% | Kay & Scarrott, 1997[136] |

| | Smoking rate [a] | | | Study details | | |
|---|---|---|---|---|---|---|
| Country | All | Male | Female | Sample size | Response rate [b] | Authors |
| United Kingdom | 5% | – | – | 557 | 70% | Allard, 2000[112] |
| United Kingdom | 6% | – | – | 49 | 79% | Newbury-Birch et al., 2002[151] |
| United Kingdom | 8% | – | – | 696 | 71% | John et al., 2003[132] |
| United Kingdom | 9% | 13% | 6% | 537 | 75% | Underwood et al., 2003[140] |
| United States | 18% | – | – | 376 | 81% | O'Shea & Corah, 1984[137] |
| United States | 8% | – | – | 630 | 8% | Christen, 1984[114] |
| United States | 8% | – | – | 1349 | 28% | Laskin, 1987[116] |
| United States | 5% | – | – | 196 | 78% | Secker-Walker et al., 1989[134] |
| United States | 6% | – | – | 1116 | 86% | Logan et al., 1992[139] |
| United States | 6% | – | – | 247 | 35% | Fried & Cohen, 1992[131] |
| United States | 2% | – | – | 462 | 73% | Hastreiter et al., 1994[138] |
| United States | 1% | – | – | 79 | 76% | Brink et al., 1994[45] |
| United States | 9% | – | – | 33 | 37% | Hill & Braithwaite, 1997[61] |
| United States | – | 6% | – | 79 | – | Merchant et al., 2002[152] |
| United States | 6% | – | – | 113 | 65% | Kenna & Wood, 2005[62] |
| United States | 6% | – | – | 391 | 53% | Tong et al., 2010[46] |
| Vietnam | 11% | – | – | 429 | 86% | An et al., 2008[41] |

[a] Smoking rates rounded to the nearest whole number, [b] Response rates rounded to the nearest whole number

## 3.3    Smoking rates among nurses

More than 80 published studies on nurses' smoking habits were located and examined for this section of the chapter, as shown in Table 3.3. Most investigations have been conducted in developed countries, with around one-third originating from the US, and around one-sixth coming from the UK. The largest study of smoking among nurses appears to have been published in 1987, in which data from almost 100,000 US nurses who had been re-cruited for the Nurses' Health Study, were analysed.[153] Follow-up data from the Nurses' Health Study were also used in the second largest investigation, published in 2004,[154] in which the results of data from 56,458 US nurses were analysed.[10, 154] Data for the third larg-est overall sample size analysed were published in 2008,[15] after data were obtained from 35,151 nurses during a New Zealand census, one of the few countries in the world which actually includes smoking-related information in their census. Aside from research proj-ects which used part of a larger national data set as their primary data source, there have also been smaller studies conducted. Some have had similarly impressive sample sizes such as an investigation of 4776 registered nurses in the Canadian Nurses Association[155] and a three-phase study of 3981 German nurses.[156]

While the number of subjects which some researchers have been recruiting may be large, not all studies have been equally impressive. Between 1976 and 2006, for example, at least nine researchers published studies where less than 100 nurses had been surveyed. The highest response rates appear to have been published in 1999 following a survey of group practices in the UK,[157] and also in 2006 as part of a larger multi-country study conducted in India and Indonesia.[90] While a 100% response rate was stated for both, this may reflect the overall small number of nurses actually surveyed by the authors.[90, 157] Nevertheless, at least three other investigations have also obtained a very high response rate of 98% when target-ing nurses in China,[158] Taiwan[159] and the US.[160] Similarly, a 97% response rate was obtained in the US,[161] and a 96% response rate was obtained during a survey of nurses in Japan.[162]

Not all studies have benefited from high response rates. At least nine nurse smoking surveys published since 1976 had obtained responses from less than half the population sampled. The lowest response rate obtained during a nurse survey appears to have been published in 1997.[163] In this study, a national nursing journal from the UK inserted lifestyle-related questionnaires into 20,000 subscription copies of their journal. At the time of publication, 1839 surveys were reported as returned (9% response rate) and the data from 1000 surveys analysed (5% of the total number originally sent out). While the small response rate was acknowledged in an editorial,[164] exactly how well their figures represent the overall nurse population or even the readership of the journal, remains unknown. From these analyses, it can be seen that the response rate, not just the overall sample size, of a tobacco smoking survey is critically important for determining how representative the data is.

Examination of the current data suggests that the overall prevalence of smoking among nurses can vary widely, both from country to country and from year to year. Some stud-ies, for example, have shown that less than 5% of nurses are smokers in China,[158,83] Hong Kong[165] and Taiwan.[159] This may reflect a cultural reluctance for women in certain parts of the world to smoke.[166, 167] At least one study from the US revealed that less than one-in-twenty nurses smoked tobacco.[161] Similarly encouraging smoking rates below 10% were recorded among nurses in the UK,[157] the US[161,168–170] and Vietnam.[41] In contrast, high contemporary smoking rates (over 40%) have been revealed in Bosnia & Herzegovina,[37] Greece,[171] Israel,[172] Italy[24, 26, 94] and Turkey.[173]

Aside from their relative epidemiological value at the time, multiple studies conducted in the same country over time may give some insight as to how smoking trends are progressing among nurses in that particular region. In this regard, tobacco consumption among Australian nurses is reported to have declined from 53% in 1976[174] to 21% in 1999,[175] while in Canada it fell from 32% in 1982[81] to 12% in 2000.[176] In the US, where a variety of smoking surveys have been performed among nurses, early research showed the smoking rate to be around 26% in the early 1980s,[177] a rate which declined to 18%[178] and then to 9%[170] by 2006. However, not all tobacco research conducted over time has revealed such clear trends in smoking reduction. In Japan, for example, the national smoking rate among female nurses was reported to be 19% in 1999.[179] In 2002, a study found that 34% of their female nurses were smoking,[180] whereas in 2006 it was reported that the rate was only 11%.[181]

In 1984, it was reported that 40% of UK nurses were tobacco smokers.[182] This rate had declined to 26% in 1992[183] and 20% in 1993.[102] Two UK publications from 2004, however,[184, 185] reported smoking rates between 17% and 26%. A more recent publication, on the other hand, reported a very high smoking rate of 35% among psychiatric nurses.[186] It is plausible that research into the demographic backgrounds of nurses in various hospitals may further explain the differences in smoking rates. To date, the only countries that have looked at smoking rates among large, comprehensive, multidisciplinary and nationally representative samples of the nursing profession appear to be Japan,[179] New Zealand[10, 11, 187] and the US.[153, 154] Further research of this nature should be conducted in other countries.

While only a small proportion of manuscripts had divided their results by gender, in some cases where it had been done, the differences in smoking rates were large. In one Chinese study, for example, the overall smoking rate was 3% but among male nurses, it was 52%.[158] Furthermore, in Japan, 75% of male nurses reported smoking, whereas only 15% of their female counterparts did.[188] Slightly higher smoking rates among male nurses were documented in Australia (56% versus 52%),[174] Japan (19% versus 11%),[181] New Zealand (20% versus 13%),[15] and the UK (17% versus 7%[189] and 47% versus 39%).[190] At least three studies, however, found that more female nurses smoked when compared to their male counterparts. In one Italian study, for example, the smoking rate was shown to be 42% among female nurses and 40% among males,[26] while in the US, it was reported that 38% of female nurses smoked but only 19% of their male counterparts did.[154] In a more recent Spanish study, the female nurse smoking rate (30%) was only slightly higher than that of male nurses (29%).[191]

Research suggests that the prevalence of smoking among nurses has varied over time. While the average smoking rate among published studies examined for this chapter was around 20%, this rate appears to be on the decline. Among manuscripts published in the mid 1970s to 1980s, for example, the average smoking rate was around 38% overall, with approximately 48% of male nurses and 40% of female nurses being smokers. Between 1986 and 1995, the overall smoking rate had declined to 21%, and then to 20% between the years 1996 to 2006. Smoking rates declined slightly differently between the genders, being 47% to 36% for males and 25% to 21% for females. Average smoking rates by country could not be reliably ascertained, simply due to the small number of studies conducted in each country (often only a single study), or the large time lag between investigations undertaken in the same countries. From the analyses undertaken for this chapter, it can be seen that the overall smoking rate among nurses has steadily declined in recent years. The quality of research on tobacco smoking within the nursing profession also appears to be improving in recent years.

Table 3.3        Smoking rates among nurses

| | Smoking rate [a] | | | Study details | | |
|---|---|---|---|---|---|---|
| Country | All | Male | Female | Sample size | Response rate [b] | Authors |
| Australia | 53% | 56% | 52% | 220 | – | Kirkby *et al.*, 1976[174] |
| Australia | 16% | – | – | 1303 | 59% | Jones *et al.*, 1998[192] |
| Australia | 21% | – | – | 1457 | 80% | Hughes & Rissel, 1999[175] |
| Australia | 22% | – | – | 335 | 88% | Nagle *et al.*, 1999[193] |
| Bosnia and Herzegovina | 51% | – | – | 97 | 81% | Hodgetts *et al.*, 2004[37] |
| Canada | 32% | – | – | 508 | – | Senior, 1982[81] |
| Canada | – | – | 23% | 822 | 90% | Dore & Hoey, 1988[194] |
| Canada | 17% | – | – | 4776 | 85% | Harrison, 1991[155] |
| Canada | 17% | – | – | 1714 | 85% | O'Connor & Harrison, 1992[195] |
| Canada | 12% | – | – | 1269 | 65% | Chalmers *et al.*, 2000[196] |
| China | 3% | 52% | – | 509 | 98% | Smith *et al.*, 2005[158] |

| | Smoking rate [a] | | | Study details | | |
|---|---|---|---|---|---|---|
| Country | All | Male | Female | Sample size | Response rate [b] | Authors |
| China | 1% | – | – | 278 | 85% | Yan *et al.*, 2008[83] |
| Denmark | 28% | – | – | 445 | 91% | Willaing *et al.*, 2003[86] |
| Denmark | 18% | – | – | 729 | 75% | Kannegaard *et al.*, 2005[87] |
| Finland | 15% | – | – | 727 | 72% | Heloma *et al.*, 1998[64] |
| Finland | 11% | – | – | 882 | 71% | Pelkonen & Kankkunen 2001[197] |
| France | 34% | – | – | 895 | 83% | Cooreman *et al.*, 1989[198] |
| Germany | 29% | – | – | 3981 | – | John & Hanke, 2003[156] |
| Greece | – | – | 46% | 114 | – | Tselebis *et al.*, 2001[199] |
| Greece | 46% | – | – | 308 | 73% | Beletsioti-Stika & Scriven, 2006[171] |
| Hong Kong | 16% | – | – | 92 | 46% | Callaghan *et al.*, 1997[200] |
| Hong Kong | 1% | – | – | 1843 | 50% | Johnston *et al.*, 2005[165] |
| India | – | – | 0% | 73 | 100% | Mohan *et al.*, 2006[90] |
| Israel | 45% | – | – | 290 | 83% | Kaplan *et al.*, 2002[172] |
| Italy | 44% | – | – | 959 | 57% | Nardini *et al.*, 1998[24] |
| Italy | 41% | 40% | 42% | 1313 | 68% | Zanetti *et al.*, 1998[26] |
| Italy | 50% | – | – | 265 | – | Ficarra *et al.*, 2010[94] |
| Japan | – | – | 19% | 2207 | 92% | Ohida *et al.*, 1999[179] |

| | Smoking rate [a] | | | Study details | | |
|---|---|---|---|---|---|---|
| Country | All | Male | Female | Sample size | Response rate [b] | Authors |
| Japan | – | 75% | 15% | 1152 | – | Ohida et al., 2000[188] |
| Japan | – | – | 34% | 1195 | 80% | Kitajima et al., 2002[180] |
| Japan | – | – | 12% | 332 | – | Ota et al., 2004[201] |
| Japan | – | – | 16% | 432 | 96% | Sekijima et al., 2005[162] |
| Japan | 11% | 19% | 11% | 860 | 74% | Smith et al., 2006[181] |
| New Zealand | – | 49% | 36% | 27,323 | – | Hay, 1980[187] |
| New Zealand | – | 39% | 31% | 30,720 | – | Hay, 1984[10] |
| New Zealand | 18% | 27% | 18% | 30,507 | – | Hay, 1998[11] |
| New Zealand | – | 20% | 13% | 35,151 | 96% | Edwards et al., 2008[15] |
| South Africa | 31% | – | – | 80 | 80% | Retief et al., 2003[202] |
| Spain | 29% | 29% | 30% | 854 | 95% | Fernandez et al., 2010[191] |
| Taiwan | – | – | 1% | 907 | 98% | Yang et al., 2001[159] |
| Turkey | 45% | – | 45% | 239 | 79% | Sezer et al., 2007[173] |
| United Kingdom | 40% | – | – | 1577 | 56% | Spencer, 1984[182] |
| United Kingdom | 21% | – | – | 663 | 70% | Davies & Rajan, 1989[47] |
| United Kingdom | – | 47% | 39% | 600 | 89% | Plant et al., 1991[190] |
| United Kingdom | 26% | – | – | 51 | 88% | Blakey & Seaton, 1992[183] |

Smoking among healthcare professionals

| | Smoking rate [a] | | | Study details | | |
| Country | All | Male | Female | Sample size | Response rate [b] | Authors |
| --- | --- | --- | --- | --- | --- | --- |
| United Kingdom | 20% | – | – | 1069 | 82% | Hussain *et al.*, 1993[102] |
| United Kingdom | 14% | – | – | 1000 | 5% | Alderman, 1997[163] |
| United Kingdom | 26% | – | – | 418 | 92% | Hope *et al.*, 1998[203] |
| United Kingdom | 7% | – | – | 58 | 100% | Steptoe *et al.*, 1999[157] |
| United Kingdom | 21% | – | – | 555 | 84% | Rowe & Clark, 1999[204] |
| United Kingdom | – | 17% | 7% | 130 | 25% | Group, 2002[189] |
| United Kingdom | 26% | – | – | 1074 | 60% | McKenna *et al.*, 2003[205] |
| United Kingdom | 17% | – | – | 167 | 39% | Dickens *et al.*, 2004[184] |
| United Kingdom | 26% | – | – | 476 | 38% | Stubbs, 2004[185] |
| United Kingdom | 35% | – | – | 92 | 58% | Bloor *et al.*, 2006[186] |
| United States | 26% | – | – | 545 | 52% | Morra & Knobf, 1983[177] |
| United States | 24% | – | – | 823 | 82% | Feldman, 1984[206] |
| United States | 22% | – | – | 1380 | 80% | Becker *et al.*, 1986[207] |
| United States | 22% | – | – | 738 | 89% | Brown & Kiss, 1987[208] |
| United States | – | – | 34% | 91,651 | – | Myers *et al.*, 1987[153] |
| United States | 20% | – | – | 499 | 70% | Haughey *et al.*, 1992[209] |
| United States | 22% | – | – | 307 | 98% | Alexander & Beck, 1990[160] |

| | Smoking rate [a] | | | Study details | | |
|---|---|---|---|---|---|---|
| Country | All | Male | Female | Sample size | Response rate [b] | Authors |
| United States | 18% | – | – | 901 | – | Nelson *et al.*, 1994[178] |
| United States | 16% | – | – | 1008 | 39% | Stillman *et al.*, 1994[210] |
| United States | 14% | – | – | 1538 | 77% | Mundt *et al.*, 1995[211] |
| United States | – | – | 20% | 952 | 19% | Blazer & Mansfield, 1995[212] |
| United States | – | – | 7% | 316 | 65% | Reeve *et al.*, 1996[168] |
| United States | 14% | – | – | 4438 | 78% | Trinkoff & Storr, 1998[213] |
| United States | – | – | 22% | 1951 | 49% | Collins *et al.*, 1999[214] |
| United States | 7% | – | – | 1508 | 38% | Sarna *et al.*, 2000[169] |
| United States | 14% | – | – | 129 | 74% | Barrett *et al.*, 2000[215] |
| United States | 13% | – | – | 98 | 94% | Borrelli *et al.*, 2001[216] |
| United States | – | – | 16% | 381 | 74% | Merchant *et al.*, 2002[152] |
| United States | 4% | – | – | 388 | 97% | Petch-Levine *et al.*, 2003[161] |
| United States | – | 19% | 38% | 56,458 | – | Bain *et al.*, 2004[154] |
| United States | 10% | – | – | 647 | 73% | Braun *et al.*, 2004[217] |
| United States | 12% | – | – | 129 | 73% | Kenna & Wood, 2005[62] |
| United States | 10% | – | – | 58 | – | Brown *et al.*, 2006[218] |

| Country | Smoking rate [a] | | | Study details | | |
|---|---|---|---|---|---|---|
| | All | Male | Female | Sample size | Response rate [b] | Authors |
| United States | 9% | – | – | 276 | 60% | Yankie et al., 2006[170] |
| United States | 13% | – | – | 388 | 70% | Tong et al., 2010[46] |
| Vietnam | 8% | – | – | 987 | 86% | An et al., 2008[41] |

[a] Smoking rates rounded to the nearest whole number, [b] Response rates rounded to the nearest whole number

# Chapter 4

# Tobacco use among healthcare students

*This chapter provides a review of international literature describing the prevalence of tobacco smoking among the students of medicine, dentistry and nursing. Results indicate that the prevalence of smoking among medical students varies widely between students of different countries, and also between male and female students within the same countries. While many cross-sectional investigations suggest that the prevalence of smoking increases as healthcare students move into the more senior grades of study, it is difficult to establish whether this trend directly reflects university seniority, increasing age, or both.*

## 4.1    Smoking rates among medical students

More than 80 published studies on smoking habits among medical students were located and examined for this section of the chapter, as shown in Table 4.1. The majority of studies had been conducted as questionnaire surveys among a complete cross-section of students within a single medical school. The next most common methodology involved surveying a single grade of medical student, often students in either the first or final year at university. The number of participants in each study ranged from 41[1] to 5744.[2] Particularly large surveys of medical students' tobacco smoking habits (where over 2000 participants were sampled) have been conducted in the US,[2, 3] Vietnam,[4] Turkey,[5] Spain[6] and Colombia.[7] Survey response rates ranged from 25%[8] to 100%.[1, 9-17] Few manuscripts had response rates below 50%,[6, 8, 18-20] while the participation rate in at least 20 studies was not specified.

After Hong Kong (1%),[19] the lowest overall prevalence rates of 2%–3% were documented in US medical schools during the late 1990s,[2, 20, 21] with similarly low levels also reported in Australia,[22] Brazil,[23] China,[24] and Uganda (3%),[25] and France[26] and India (4%).[27] Smoking rates below 10% of the medical student population were shown to occur in Australia (4%–6%),[28-31] Canada (6%),[32] China (6%),[33] India (7%),[34] Thailand (7%),[35] the US (5%–7%),[18, 36] Egypt (8%),[25] and Malaysia[17, 37] and Pakistan (9%).[38] In contrast, high smoking rates (>35%) among medical students have been recorded in Albania (43%),[25] Greece (41%),[39] Croatia (37%),[25] Spain (37%),[40] Hungary (36%)[41] and the Slovak Republic (36%).[42] Marked differences in smoking rates were reported by gender in almost all studies, with male students generally associated with the higher rates. From the published literature, it appears that the international prevalence of tobacco smoking among male medical students ranges from 1% in Hong Kong[19] to 65% in Albania.[25] Other relatively high prevalence rates among male medical students were also documented in Japan (51%–58%),[10, 11] Vietnam (44%),[4] Spain (42%),[6] Greece (41%)[39] and Italy (40%).[43]

The smoking prevalence rate among female students was generally lower than their male counterparts at the same medical school across a range of studies, and at least nine investigations reported not having any female smokers at all. This particular phenomenon was seen among research conducted in China,[33, 44] India,[14, 27] Malaysia,[17, 37] Saudi Arabia,[45] Uganda[25] and Thailand.[35] It has been previously suggested that smoking may be regarded as inappropriate behaviour for women in certain countries.[46, 47] Nevertheless, it is also possible that some females who did actually smoke in these countries may not have admitted their smoking habit during the survey for similar reasons. Aside from countries where the smoking prevalence among female medical students was reported to be either zero or was not recorded at all, very low smoking prevalence rates of only 1% have been documented among female students in China,[24] Egypt,[25] Hong Kong,[19] Malaysia,[16] Pakistan[38, 48, 49] and Tunisia.[50]

One of the most important issues for smoking research among university students is to what extent tobacco usage increases as a student progresses. For the current chapter, a number of studies were located that had been conducted among a cross-section of students at the same medical school. Almost all reported that tobacco smoking rates among medical students tend to increase between the year of entry and the final year. In an Indian study, for example, the smoking prevalence ranged from 7% among male first-year students to 16% among fifth-year students.[27] In another study from India, smoking rates increased from 17% to 43% between the first and fifth years, respectively.[51] Research conducted in the UK documented a prevalence rate rising from 16% among first-year students to 20% among fifth-year students.[52] Similarly in Serbia, smoking rates were shown to have increased from 27% to 36% during the five years of medical school.[53] Despite these findings, however, not all studies of tobacco usage among medical students have demonstrated a trend of increasing prevalence by year of study. In Iran,[8] for example, it has been reported that tobacco usage ranged from 18% in the first-year group, to 7% in the third-year group and then back up to 17% in the fourth-year group. Considering the results of previous investigations and the fact that response rates were not mentioned, the possibility of demographic differences in the third-year group of the Iranian study[8] cannot be discounted.

Aside from point-prevalence surveys of tobacco smoking, several longitudinal studies of tobacco smoking have also been conducted among medical students in Australia,[29] India,[34, 54] Ireland,[55] Japan,[56] Malaysia[37] and Turkey.[57] Results from these investigations are worthy of some interpretation. In the Australian investigation,[29] three separate groups of male and female students in their fifth-year of study at medical school were targeted. Surveys were conducted in 1986, 1990 and 1993, with response rates of 65%, 73% and 68%, respectively. The prevalence of smoking among students steadily declined over the eight-year period, beginning at 10% in 1986, falling to 4% in 1990 and then to 3% in 1993.[29] In another study,[54] 10 successive groups of male students enrolled at an Indian medical school between 1955 and 1988 were investigated. Similar to the previously mentioned Australian study,[29] the Indian researchers reported that the overall prevalence of smoking among medical students was in decline, falling from 42% (in the period 1955–60) to 25% (in the period 1985–88).[54] Additionally, three separate groups of male and female students were followed through an Irish medical school between 1973 and 2002.[55] The 1973 investigation targeted students in their first, third, fourth and sixth year of study, while in 1990 and 2002, all six years of the medical school were surveyed. The overall prevalence of smoking declined from 29% in 1973, to 15% in 1990 and then 10% in 2002.[55] A Malaysian study[37] recruited a cohort of male and female medical students in their first year of study during 1991–92, following them up two years later in the 1993–94 school year. Unlike the three previous investigations, the prevalence of smoking among this Malaysian cohort actually increased from 9% to 11% during the follow-up period.[37]

A recently published longitudinal study of tobacco smoking among medical students was undertaken in Turkey,[57] and in this investigation 22% of students (male and female) were smoking in their first-year of study, a rate which had risen to 27% by the sixth year. Approximately one-third of non-smokers in the first-year of study had become smokers by the end of their 6th year at medical school.[57] While it would have been useful to compare the smoking habits of undergraduate medical students with postgraduate medical students, few if any researchers appear to have done so.

Table 4.1        Smoking rates among medical students

| | Smoking rate [a] | | | Study details | | |
| --- | --- | --- | --- | --- | --- | --- |
| Country | All | Male | Female | Sample size | Response rate [b] | Authors |
| Albania | 14% | 34% | 5% | 149 | 82% | Vakeflliu et al., 2002[58] |
| Albania | 43% | 65% | 36% | 114 | – | CDC, 2005[25] |
| Argentina | 36% | 33% | 37% | 296 | – | CDC, 2005[25] |
| Australia | 6% | – | – | 431 | – | Engs, 1980[28] |
| Australia | 4% | – | – | 250 | 79% | Roche & Beauchamp, 1994[30] |
| Australia | 4% | – | – | 173 | 79% | Roche et al., 1996[59] |
| Australia | 3% | – | – | 594 | 79% | Richmond & Kehoe, 1997[22] |
| Australia | 5% | – | – | 379 | 69% | Roche, 1997[60] |
| Brazil | 14% | 10% | 18% | 103 | 96% | Paine et al., 1985[61] |

| | Smoking rate [a] | | | Study details | | |
|---|---|---|---|---|---|---|
| Country | All | Male | Female | Sample size | Response rate [b] | Authors |
| Brazil | 3% | – | – | 513 | 73% | Daudt et al., 1999[23] |
| Brazil | 17% | – | – | 316 | 99% | Stramari et al., 2009[62] |
| Canada | 6% | – | – | 175 | 54% | Thakore et al., 2009[32] |
| China | 3% | 6% | 1% | 1392 | 86% | Lei et al., 1997[24] |
| China | – | 38% | 0% | 1540 | 96% | Xiang et al., 1999[44] |
| China | 6% | 13% | 0% | 207 | 92% | Smith et al., 2005[33] |
| Colombia | 26% | 28% | 24% | 2021 | 90% | Rosselli et al., 2001[7] |
| Croatia | 29% | – | – | 775 | 98% | Trkulja et al., 2003[63] |
| Croatia | 37% | 36% | 37% | 377 | – | CDC, 2005[25] |
| Egypt | 8% | 13% | 1% | 1749 | – | CDC, 2005[25] |
| France | 4% | – | – | 136 | – | Franca et al., 2010[26] |
| Germany | 24% | 29% | 18% | 696 | 85% | Brenner & Scharrer, 1996[64] |
| Germany | 25% | 32% | 22% | 258 | 87% | Kusma et al., 2010[65] |
| Greece | – | 33% | 28% | 849 | 98% | Mammas et al., 2003[66] |
| Greece | 41% | 41% | 40% | 1072 | – | Sichletidis et al., 2006[39] |
| Greece | 35% | – | – | 269 | – | Alexopoulos et al., 2010[67] |
| Hong Kong | 1% | 1% | 1% | 305 | 45% | Lam et al., 2009[19] |
| Hungary | 21% | – | – | 177 | 73% | Piko et al., 1996[70] |
| Hungary | 36% | – | – | 91 | 90% | Piko, 2002[41] |

| | Smoking rate [a] | | | Study details | | |
|---|---|---|---|---|---|---|
| Country | All | Male | Female | Sample size | Response rate [b] | Authors |
| India | – | 3% | 0% | 705 | 100% | Roy & Chakraborty, 1981[14] |
| India | 11% | – | – | 672 | 90% | Singh *et al.*, 1981[71] |
| India | 27% | – | – | 1600 | 80% | Sandell *et al.*, 1983[72] |
| India | 7% | – | – | 355 | – | Behera & Malik, 1987[34] |
| India | 31% | 35% | 5% | 854 | 66% | Singh *et al.*, 1989[51] |
| India | – | 19% | – | 196 | 64% | Venkataraman *et al.*, 1996[54] |
| India | – | 23% | – | 400 | 93% | Sinha & Gupta, 2001[73] |
| India | 4% | 5% | 0% | 1189 | 74% | Ramakrishna *et al.*, 2005[27] |
| India | – | 8% | – | 1130 | 75% | Mohan *et al.*, 2006[74] |
| India | 12% | – | – | 1117 | 89% | Sinha *et al.*, 2010[75] |
| Iran | 13% | – | – | 421 | 25% | Ahmadi *et al.*, 2001[8] |
| Ireland | 10% | 10% | 8% | 537 | 94% | Boland *et al.*, 2006[55] |
| Italy | 30% | 40% | 25% | 200 | 94% | Melani *et al.*, 2000[43] |
| Italy | 35% | – | – | 60 | – | Ficarra *et al.*, 2010[76] |
| Japan | – | 51% | 8% | 129 | 100% | Kawane, 1987[10] |
| Japan | – | 58% | – | 77 | 100% | Kawane, 1992[11] |
| Japan | 17% | – | – | 100 | 100% | Kusunoki *et al.*, 1999[12] |
| Japan | – | 16% | 4% | 1366 | – | Ozasa *et al.*, 2005[56] |

| | Smoking rate [a] | | | Study details | | |
|---|---|---|---|---|---|---|
| Country | All | Male | Female | Sample size | Response rate [b] | Authors |
| Japan | 14% | 18% | 5% | 1619 | 88% | Tamaki *et al.*, 2010[77] |
| Jordan | 12% | 26% | 7% | 340 | 100% | Merrill *et al.*, 2009[13] |
| Kenya | 21% | – | – | 181 | – | Komu *et al.*, 2009[78] |
| Malaysia | 10% | 17% | 1% | 271 | 100% | Wong & Chen, 1989[16] |
| Malaysia | 9% | 22% | 0% | 395 | 100% | Yaacob & Abdullah, 1994[17] |
| Malaysia | 9% | – | 0% | 148 | 95% | Frisch *et al.*, 1999[37] |
| Netherlands | 27% | 31% | 23% | 725 | 95% | Waalkens *et al.*, 1992[68] |
| Netherlands | 18% | 19% | 16% | 160 | 80% | Dekker *et al.*, 1993[69] |
| Pakistan | – | 21% | 1% | 1363 | 62% | Ahmed & Jafarey, 1983[48] |
| Pakistan | 11% | 17% | 4% | 289 | 89% | Hussain *et al.*, 1995[79] |
| Pakistan | – | 26% | 2% | 264 | 92% | Omair *et al.*, 2002[80] |
| Pakistan | 14% | 22% | 4% | 271 | 90% | Khan *et al.*, 2005[81] |
| Pakistan | 15% | 32% | 1% | 165 | 84% | Mubeen *et al.*, 2008[49] |
| Pakistan | 20% | – | – | 974 | – | Khan et al., 2008[82] |
| Pakistan | 9% | 23% | 1% | 1529 | 85% | Minhas & Rahman, 2009[38] |
| Saudi Arabia | – | 33% | – | 414 | 100% | Jarallah, 1992[9] |
| Saudi Arabia | – | 13% | – | 322 | 81% | Al-Turki, 2006[83] |

| | Smoking rate [a] | | | Study details | | |
|---|---|---|---|---|---|---|
| Country | All | Male | Female | Sample size | Response rate [b] | Authors |
| Saudi Arabia | 19% | 24% | 0% | 215 | 65% | Al-Haqwi *et al.*, 2010[45] |
| Serbia | 31% | 36% | 28% | 1657 | 54% | Vlajinac *et al.*, 1989[53] |
| Serbia | 18% | 16% | 24% | 187 | – | CDC, 2005[25] |
| Slovak Republic | 36% | – | – | 185 | 98% | Kavcova *et al.*, 2004[42] |
| Spain | 44% | 42% | 45% | 2308 | 40% | Rodriguez & Cami, 1986[6] |
| Spain | 37% | – | – | 41 | 100% | Moreno San-Pedro *et al.*, 2006[1] |
| Syria | 11% | 16% | 3% | 570 | 93% | Almerie *et al.*, 2008[84] |
| Thailand | 7% | – | 0% | 256 | – | Songkla & Saenghirun-vattana, 1985[35] |
| Tunisia | 19% | 30% | 1% | 230 | 74% | Harrabi *et al.*, 2006[50] |
| Turkey | – | 31% | 10% | 3073 | 88% | Kocabas *et al.*, 1994[5] |
| Turkey | 32% | 39% | 22% | 447 | – | Akvardar *et al.*, 2003[85] |
| Turkey | 33% | – | – | 690 | 89% | Gulec *et al.*, 2005[86] |
| Turkey | 22% | 28% | 10% | 126 | 98% | Senol *et al.*, 2006[57] |
| Uganda | 3% | 4% | 0% | 151 | – | CDC, 2005[25] |
| United Kingdom | 35% | – | – | 134 | – | Birkner & Kunze, 1978[87] |
| United Kingdom | 17% | 18% | 15% | 1112 | 96% | Elkind, 1982[52] |
| United Kingdom | – | 12% | 30% | 186 | 99% | Ashton & Kamali, 1995[88] |
| United Kingdom | – | 23% | 17% | 566 | – | Engs & Van Teijlingen, 1997[89] |

| | Smoking rate [a] | | | Study details | | |
|---|---|---|---|---|---|---|
| Country | All | Male | Female | Sample size | Response rate [b] | Authors |
| United Kingdom | – | 18% | 14% | 785 | 100% | Webb *et al.*, 1998[15] |
| United States | 14% | – | – | 238 | 97% | Birkner & Kunze, 1978[87] |
| United States | 5% | – | – | 589 | 41% | Conard *et al.*, 1988[18] |
| United States | 10% | – | – | 2046 | 67% | Baldwin *et al.*, 1991[3] |
| United States | 7% | – | – | 105 | 50% | Najem *et al.*, 1995[36] |
| United States | 2% | – | – | 5744 | – | Sockrider *et al.*, 1998[2] |
| United States | 2% | 3% | 2% | 548 | 55% | Mangus *et al.*, 1998[21] |
| United States | 3% | – | – | 397 | 48% | Patkar *et al.*, 2003[20] |
| Vietnam | 25% | 44% | 2% | 4701 | 99% | Huy *et al.*, 2008[4] |

[a] Smoking rates rounded to the nearest whole number, [b] Response rates rounded to the nearest whole number

## 4.2    Smoking rates among dental students

More than 30 published studies on smoking habits of dental students were located and examined for this section of the chapter, as shown in Table 4.2. Sample sizes of the surveys ranged from 27[78] to 1499.[75] Although one Romanian study recruited a relatively large overall group of 1387 students,[90] only 94 were from the dental faculty. Response rates ranged from 62%[91] to 100%,[92] except for 20 studies where the response rate was unspecified and four studies where students were recruited from multiple faculties.[36, 90, 93, 94] When considered from an international perspective, the overall prevalence of smoking among dental students is relatively low in Australia (2%),[95] Canada (3%),[96] the US (4%),[97] Brazil (6%)[93] and the UK (7%).[98] Other areas such as India (10%)[25] and Kenya (11%)[78] also reported smoking rates that were well below 20%. This encouraging trend was not uniform, however, with almost half the dental students in Greece (47%),[99] Serbia (43%)[25] and Romania (38%),[100] and roughly one-third of those in Hungary (34%),[94] Pakistan (34%),[82] France (33%)[101] and Albania (30%)[25] being smokers. Some of the earliest smoking research among the dental student demographic was conducted in the early 1970s in the US,[102, 103] Norway and India.[104] At the time, it was reported that 35% of US dental students were smokers,[103] a rate which had decreased to 11% in 1995[36] and then to 4% by 2004.[97] Similarly, UK dental student smoking rates decreased from 50% in 1965[105] to 7% in 2006.[98] Furthermore, India and Canada also appeared to experience a similar decrease, with their dental student smoking rates falling from 23% in 1970[104] to 10% in 2005,[25] and from 8% in 1981[106] to 3% in 1997,[96] respectively. Time-related trends for tobacco smoking among dental students in other regions are more difficult to ascertain however, due to the lack of multiple studies conducted in the same country over time. Interestingly, the smoking rate among dental students in Romania appears to have remained relatively unchanged between 1986 (39%)[90] and 2007 (37%).[100]

Where smoking rates were provided by gender, male dental students for the most part appear to smoke at higher rates than females. In Bangladesh, for example, 47% of male dental students smoked but only 3% of females did so.[25] Similar contrasts were also reported in Japan (33% versus 7%),[107] Jordan (31% versus 4%),[108, 109] India (15% versus 2%),[25] Saudi Arabia (13% versus 2%)[110] and Tunisia (14% versus 4%).[111] These findings may suggest a cultural reluctance for females to smoke in certain parts of the world, such as Asia and the Middle East. In contrast, in Greece, for example,[99] 51% of female students smoked compared to 43% of males. A similar situation was also reported in Serbia,[25] where the tobacco smoking rates were 47% and 30%, respectively. However, half the studies examined for this chapter did not divide their smoking prevalence rates by sex, making it impossible to undertake any further gender comparisons.

The prevalence of smoking among dental students may also vary by year of study in the dentistry course. During one investigation from the UK, for example,[112] 4% of the males and 1% of the female students in their first three years of study were smokers. This rate had risen to 21% and 13% respectively, among students in their fourth or fifth year. A longitudinal study from the UK followed a single year cohort of dental students from their second year to their fifth and final year of study.[113] During this time, their smoking prevalence rate appeared to decline from 11% to 5%. The results of a longitudinal investigation of French undergraduate dental students[101] are a little more difficult to decipher however, and as such, it is premature to surmise whether these changes in smoking prevalence represent a genuine trend for the demographic.

Despite some variations in the apparent epidemiological quality of smoking research previously conducted among dental students, a large proportion of all investigations we reviewed had reasonable sample sizes and sufficiently high response rates. This in turn, affords a high degree of confidence in the data presented. The philosophical validity of comparing the demographic items of dental students from one country to the next has been described elsewhere, both in the affirmative.[104, 114] From a global perspective, the overall findings from this chapter suggest that tobacco smoking is becoming steadily less common among dental students in Australia, Canada, the UK and the US. This is not surprising, however, as it has previously been noted that dentists generally smoke at one of the lowest rates among all health professionals, and much lower than that of the communities in which they live.[115] Somewhat discouragingly, it does appear that smoking remains quite common among dental students in certain other regions such as Greece,[99] Romania,[100] Serbia,[25] Hungary,[94] Pakistan,[82] France,[101] and Albania.[25]

The identification of year of study in the dentistry course as a possible confounder was also an interesting observation. A greater awareness of the negative health effects related to smoking among more senior dental students may offer a possible explanation for such behaviour, although it is not clear exactly who is more likely to smoke among dental students – the junior or senior students. Exactly why fewer dental students in some countries appear to be smoking tobacco when compared to others remains unclear, although it may reflect similar social issues to those experienced by medical students.[116] There are believed to be certain demographic and professional similarities between dentists and physicians, with physicians in most societies tending to give up smoking before the general population.[117] Dentists probably do so for similar reasons. Even so, the exact situation is still unclear among dental students around the world, and further smoking research will be needed to help elucidate these issues in future.

Table 4.2        Smoking rates among dental students

| | Smoking rate [a] | | | Study details | | |
|---|---|---|---|---|---|---|
| Country | All | Male | Female | Sample size | Response rate [b] | Authors |
|---|---|---|---|---|---|---|
| Albania | 30% | 38% | 27% | 41 | – | CDC, 2005[25] |
| Australia | 13% | – | – | 248 | 88% | Rikard-Bell *et al.*, 2003[118] |
| Australia | 2% | – | – | 56 | – | Smith *et al.*, 2009[95] |
| Bangladesh | 22% | 47% | 3% | 192 | – | CDC, 2005[25] |
| Brazil | 6% | – | – | – | – | de Andrade *et al.*, 2006[93] |
| Canada | 8% | – | – | 73 | – | Ashley, 1981[106] |
| Canada | 7% | – | – | 140 | 94% | Hussey *et al.*, 1990[119] |
| Canada | 3% | – | – | 120 | – | Tarlo *et al.*, 1997[96] |
| France | 33% | – | – | 1192 | 99% | Hennequin *et al.*, 2002[101] |
| Greece | 47% | 43% | 51% | 165 | 98% | Polychon-opoulou, *et al.*, 2004[99] |
| Hungary | 34% | – | – | – | – | Nagy *et al.*, 2004[94] |

| | Smoking rate [a] | | | Study details | | |
|---|---|---|---|---|---|---|
| Country | All | Male | Female | Sample size | Response rate [b] | Authors |
| India | 23% | – | – | 230 | – | Johansen, 1970[104] |
| India | 10% | 15% | 2% | 1266 | – | CDC, 2005[25] |
| India | 10% | – | – | 1499 | 93% | Sinha *et al.*, 2010[75] |
| Iran | 23% | – | – | 263 | 100% | Khami *et al.*, 2010[92] |
| Ireland | 20% | 21% | 19% | 278 | 76% | McCartan *et al.*, 1993[120] |
| Israel | 17% | 21% | 13% | 275 | 99% | Vered *et al.*, 2010[121] |
| Japan | 22% | 33% | 7% | 320 | 91% | Sugiura *et al.*, 2005[107] |
| Jordan | 17% | 31% | 4% | 314 | 84% | Al-Omari & Hamasha, 2005;[109] Al-Omari *et al.*, 2006[108] |
| Kenya | 11% | – | – | 27 | – | Komu *et al.*, 2009[78] |
| Netherlands | 24% | – | – | 375 | 62% | Plasschaert *et al.*, 2001[91] |
| Norway | 24% | – | – | 70 | – | Johansen, 1970[104] |
| Pakistan | 34% | – | – | 230 | – | Khan *et al.*, 2008[82] |
| Romania | 39% | – | – | 94 | – | Ionescu & Mihaescu, 1986[90] |
| Romania | 37% | 52% | 32% | 290 | 92% | Dumitrescu, 2007[100] |
| Saudi Arabia | – | 13% | 2% | 372 | 77% | Almas *et al.*, 2003[110] |
| Serbia | 43% | 30% | 47% | 152 | – | CDC, 2005[25] |
| South Africa | 24% | 33% | 17% | 302 | – | Gordon & Rayner, 2010[122] |
| Tunisia | 18% | 14% | 4% | 140 | – | Maatouk *et al.*, 2006[111] |

Smoking among healthcare professionals

| | Smoking rate [a] | | | Study details | | |
| Country | All | Male | Female | Sample size | Response rate [b] | Authors |
| --- | --- | --- | --- | --- | --- | --- |
| United Kingdom | 50% | 58% | 43% | 106 | – | Curson & Manson, 1965[105] |
| United Kingdom | 13% | – | – | 96 | 91% | Hussey et al., 1990[119] |
| United Kingdom | – | 4% | 1% | 200 | 76% | Underwood & Fox, 2000 (Years 1–3)[112] |
| United Kingdom | – | 21% | 13% | 200 | 76% | Underwood & Fox, 2000 (Years 4–5)[112] |
| United Kingdom | 11% | – | – | 47 | 71% | Newbury-Birch et al., 2002 (Year 2)[113] |
| United Kingdom | 5% | – | – | 53 | 80% | Newbury-Birch et al., 2002 (Year 5)[113] |
| United Kingdom | 7% | – | – | 218 | 83% | Barber & Fairclough, 2006[98] |
| United Kingdom | – | 27% | 14% | 258 | 67% | Underwood et al., 2010[123] |
| United States | 35% | – | – | 401 | – | Olson et al., 1970[103] |
| United States | 31% | – | – | 204 | – | Olson & Shapiro, 1971 (Years 1–2)[102] |
| United States | 40% | – | – | 197 | – | Olson & Shapiro, 1971 (Years 3–4)[102] |
| United States | 11% | – | – | 148 | – | Najem et al., 1995[36] |
| United States | 20% | – | – | 244 | 81% | Yip et al., 2000[124] |
| United States | 4% | – | – | 139 | 99% | Victoroff et al., 2004[97] |

[a] Smoking rates rounded to the nearest whole number, [b] Response rates rounded to the nearest whole number

## 4.3   Smoking rates among nursing students

More than 30 published studies on smoking habits among nursing students were located and examined for this section of the chapter, as shown in Table 4.3. The overall prevalence of smoking among nursing students appears to vary widely. In Iran,[125] for example, only 3% of nursing students were revealed as smokers, whereas in Israel[126] and Greece,[127] smoking rates were 22% and 36% respectively; even though all three studies were conducted in the same year. Interestingly, two Japanese investigations have also documented wide variations in prevalence, reporting a very low smoking rate of only 6%,[128] and a four times higher level of 24%[129] in the same year. Possible reasons for the discrepancy may relate to the different demographics from which their samples were sourced; that is, the inherent differences between students who study nursing at a vocational college or those who study at universities. Either way, both Japanese studies revealed that smoking prevalence increased by year of study, with students in the senior grades smoking at higher rates than their junior colleagues. In the US, postgraduate nursing students were found to smoke at higher rates when compared to undergraduates.[36] Based on the findings of cross-sectional studies alone, it is difficult to ascertain whether smoking actually increases or decreases by year of study in a nursing course.

Seniority in a nursing course was not the only complexity encountered during the examination of material for this section of the chapter. In one study from Scotland, for example,[130] a small proportion of nursing students believed smoking was not very harmful to health. Similarly in a Greek study, it was revealed that smoking was actually more common among nursing students with asthma when compared to their non-asthmatic classmates, and that the overall smoking rate among nursing students was quite high (36%).[127] The highest contemporary smoking rates were reported among students in Italy (51%),[131,132] Hungary (48%) [41] and the UK (43%),[133] where roughly half of those surveyed were current tobacco users. In some studies, nursing students' smoking habits have been shown to be associated with gender[125, 126] and other demographic factors.[126] A student's potential role in helping their patients to quit may also be controversial, as only one quarter of nursing students believed medical smoking cessations would be effective.[131]

Surveying one or two grades of student appears to be the most common method for investigating tobacco smoking rates. Many single-grade studies revealed some interesting information with regard to students' personal smoking habits. In an Australian study,[134] most students had actually begun smoking before entering their nursing school. In a Canadian study, however,[135] having friends who smoked was revealed as an important reason for commencing the habit, while a US study demonstrated that tension relief was the main reason for smoking.[136] Exposure to cigarette advertising may represent another potential initiation factor for nursing students, and in this regard, a Japanese study has reported that students were frequently exposed to cigarette advertising in many different formats.[137] Student nurses may also have some confusion regarding their potential status as role models for appropriate behaviour.[138] In Australia, for example,[139] a study of hospital-based student nurses demonstrated that they were unconvinced about the health promotion role of nurses, while in the US,[140] nurses who were smokers were less likely to participate in tobacco control activities.

Although longitudinal studies represent an accurate method for determining the progression of smoking trends over time (particularly causation), similar to medical and dental students, very few investigations of this nature appear to have been conducted among nursing students. Researchers may be reluctant to begin such studies due to a potentially high dropout rate among nursing students as they work through their degree, a potentially high attrition rate for the follow up component, as well as other issues relating to ethical concerns and privacy issues when individuals have to be specifically re-contacted over a number of years. Some longitudinal studies of students at Japanese nursing universities and vocational nursing schools reported that the prevalence of smoking increased by 10% at the vocational schools and 3% at the universities.[141] The authors achieved high follow-up rates of 84% and 81% respectively, suggesting that response bias was minimised. A similar increase in smoking was reported in a US[142] study which followed a second-year cohort of university students over two years and found that the prevalence of smoking had increased by 2% during this time. The US study benefited from a high follow-up rate (80%) although the total number of subjects in the final group was limited (less than 60 remained by follow-up). In Italy, a study followed over 500 first-year students for two years and found that their smoking prevalence had increased by 7% during the study period – with over half of the university-based nursing students being smokers by the end of the course.[143] In a longitudinal study of health behaviours (not only smoking) from Canada, a first year cohort of university students was followed over three years and it was found that their smoking rate actually decreased by 2%, falling from 12% to 10%.[144] The results of this study cannot be generalised, however, as the final follow-up group consisted of only 52 students from the original total of 193, a follow-up rate of less than 30%.

Despite the fact that many nursing students continue to smoke, few researchers have undertaken intervention studies among this group. In Denmark, for example,[145] 220 students (of whom 18% were smokers) were recruited in a study which administered eight lectures on the health consequences of smoking. The authors utilised a controlled study design, where participants were randomly allocated into either the intervention or control group. By the follow-up period seven weeks later however, no change in smoking rates was observed. A study from the UK (Northern Ireland) conducted as a one-year smoking intervention among a small group of nursing students[146] consisted of individualised counselling based on the specific needs of each student. By the follow-up period one year later, 25% of smokers had quit. The relative value of this intervention should be treated with caution however, as participants were initially required to have 'expressed a desire to give up smoking'. Furthermore, participants were assigned to either the intervention program or comparison group 'based on their preferences'.[146] This suggests that students who did not wish to give up smoking were not included in the study, while students who preferred interventions were subsequently assigned to the intervention group. It is possible, therefore, that the 25% reduction in smoking rates observed at follow-up may reflect a 25% effectiveness rate among students who already wanted to quit smoking. This is not to say that smoking interventions are not effective or should not be attempted, rather it is the overall subgroup of smokers among nursing students who should be targeted for aggressive intervention. In another study from Ireland, a series of passive interventions and stress discussion groups were undertaken with nursing students, among whom 34% were smokers.[147] Three years later, no significant change in smoking prevalence was observed during the follow-up, although there was an increase in the number of students who participated in regular exercise (another variable investigated during the study).

Table 4.3           Smoking rates among nursing students

| Country | Smoking rate [a] | | | Study details | | |
|---|---|---|---|---|---|---|
| | All | Male | Female | Sample size | Response rate [b] | Authors |
| Albania | 42% | 58% | 36% | 271 | – | CDC, 2005[25] |
| Australia | 39% | – | – | 292 | – | Neil *et al.*, 1980[148] |
| Australia | 65% | – | – | 72 | – | Adams *et al.*, 1994 (hospital)[139] |
| Australia | 45% | – | – | 95 | – | Adams *et al.*, 1994 (tertiary)[139] |
| Australia | 24% | 19% | 25% | 366 | 86% | Clark *et al.*, 2004[134] |
| Australia | 16% | 15% | 16% | 274 | 85% | Smith & Leggat, 2007[149] |
| Bosnia/ Herzegovina | 33% | 27% | 35% | 791 | – | CDC, 2005[25] |
| Brazil | 7% | – | – | – | – | de Andrade *et al.*, 2006[93] |
| Canada | 24% | – | – | 914 | 80% | O'Connor & Harrison, 1992[135] |
| Canada | 13% | – | – | 272 | 62% | Chalmers *et al.*, 2003[138] |
| France | 17% | – | – | 248 | – | Franca *et al.*, 2010[26] |
| Greece | 36% | – | – | 268 | 98% | Krommydas *et al.*, 2004[127] |
| Hungary | 48% | – | – | 100 | 90% | Piko, 2002[41] |

| | Smoking rate [a] | | | Study details | | |
|---|---|---|---|---|---|---|
| Country | All | Male | Female | Sample size | Response rate [b] | Authors |
| India | 3% | – | – | 1082 | 93% | Sinha *et al.*, 2010[75] |
| Iran | 3% | 15% | 1% | 400 | 93% | Ahmadi *et al.*, 2004[125] |
| Ireland | 34% | – | – | 169 | – | Hope *et al.*, 1998[147] |
| Israel | 22% | 30% | 20% | 782 | 69% | Baron-Epel *et al.*, 2004[126] |
| Italy | 51% | – | – | 662 | 88% | Boccoli *et al.*, 1996[131] |
| Italy | 43% | 49% | 42% | 205 | 88% | Melani *et al.*, 2000[43] |
| Italy | 51% | 60% | 48% | 252 | 92% | Melani *et al.*, 2001[132] |
| Italy | – | 43% | 33% | 505 | 99% | Zanetti *et al.*, 2003[150] |
| Italy | 44% | 53% | 39% | 812 | 87% | Biraghi & Tortorano, 2010[151] |
| Japan | 18% | – | – | 197 | 100% | Sone, 1997[137] |
| Japan | – | – | 25% | 3866 | 93% | Ohida *et al.*, 2001 (nursing)[152] |
| Japan | – | – | 13% | 539 | 91% | Ohida *et al.*, 2001 (public health)[152] |
| Japan | – | – | 22% | 325 | 95% | Ohida *et al.*, 2001 (mid-wifery)[152] |
| Japan | 24% | – | – | 3866 | 93% | Suzuki, Ohida *et al.*, 2005[129] |
| Japan | 6% | – | – | 716 | 96% | Sekijima *et al.*, 2005[128] |
| Kenya | 15% | – | – | 20 | – | Komu *et al.*, 2009[78] |

| | Smoking rate [a] | | | Study details | | |
| Country | All | Male | Female | Sample size | Response rate [b] | Authors |
| --- | --- | --- | --- | --- | --- | --- |
| Turkey | 29% | – | – | 253 | 84% | Durmaz & Üstün, 2006[153] |
| Uganda | 1% | 3% | <1% | 378 | – | CDC, 2005[25] |
| United Kingdom | 36% | – | – | 563 | 100% | Booth & Faulkner, 1986[154] |
| United Kingdom | 43% | – | – | 350 | 95% | Carmichael & Cockcroft, 1990[133] |
| United Kingdom | 33% | – | – | 649 | 95% | Blakey & Seaton, 1992[130] |
| United Kingdom | 34% | – | – | 146 | 58% | West & Hargreaves, 1995[155] |
| United Kingdom | 28% | – | – | 96 | 72% | Charlton et al., 1997[156] |
| United States | 30% | – | – | 1153 | 45% | Haughey et al., 1986[157] |
| United States | 11% | – | – | 229 | 45% | Najem et al., 1995[36] |
| United States | 24% | – | – | 476 | 89% | Gorin, 2001[140] |
| United States | 6% | – | – | 200 | 47% | Jenkins & Ahijevych, 2003[136] |
| United States | 14% | – | – | 126 | 50% | Patkar et al., 2003[20] |

[a] Smoking rates rounded to the nearest whole number, [b] Response rates rounded to the nearest whole number

# Chapter 5

# Success stories in declining tobacco use

*This chapter describes two success stories in tobacco control among healthcare professionals: the decline of smoking among doctors in Australia and the US during the mid to late 20th century. The published literature on this topic documents a continuous reduction in smoking rates among Australian doctors since the 1960s, with a similar trend also seen among their counterparts in the US. Overall, this chapter suggests that not only do very few Australian and American doctors smoke when compared to their counterparts internationally, but also that an active professional community can make a positive difference to the lifestyle choices of its members.*

## 5.1　Smoking rates among Australian doctors

More than 10 studies have investigated tobacco-smoking habits among Australian doctors, as shown in Table 5.1. All were conducted as self-reporting postal surveys, with the earliest being in 1964[1] and the most recent conducted in 1997.[2] Five investigations sourced their participants from lists of registered medical practitioners, two involved surveys sent to readers of a specific journal, two studies recruited doctors who were enrolled in postgraduate training programs, one study targeted doctors on a commercial mailing list, while the recruitment method of the remaining investigation was not clearly specified. Response rates ranged from 14%[3, 4] to 80%,[5] with most above 50%.[2, 4–9] Almost one-third of Australian doctors were smoking in the 1960s,[1] although by the early 1980s this rate had declined to one-in-ten and continued a downward trend in later years. By the 1990s, only one-in-twenty doctors reported to be smokers. The two most recent surveys suggest that smoking is now very rare among Australian doctors, with less than 5% being current smokers.[2, 6] The proportion of Australian doctors who reported themselves as non-smokers or ex-smokers has slowly increased over time. In 1964, for example,[1] half the respondents surveyed were non-smokers, a rate which had risen dramatically by 1982.[10] The proportion of Australian doctors who had quit smoking also appeared to rise during this period, from 18% in 1964 to 38% between 1970 and 1974.

Over a similar time period, the percentage of Australian doctors engaging in anti-smoking counselling also appeared to improve dramatically. In 1964, for example,[1] less than half the doctors surveyed (39%) were actively advising their patients not to smoke. By 1982, however, 91% of doctors reported that they were counselling patients in this regard.[10] As with most countries, the intrinsic dangers of tobacco smoking were almost universally recognised by Australian doctors in the mid to late 20th century. In 1964, 96% of Australian doctors believed that cigarette smoking was a health hazard.[1] The proportion of affirmative responses to this question had increased to 98% by 1970. These results suggest that doctors who continued to smoke after 1970 (over 10% of the group) were no doubt aware of the personal health hazards they faced.[11]

Although smoking rates among Australian doctors have clearly declined in recent years, it is not clear whether they are doing enough to stop their patients smoking.[12] It has been suggested that doctors are not always successful in recognising which of their patients actually smoke, with a study of Australian general practitioners, for example,[13] finding that only 56% of patients who smoked were correctly identified as such. Additional work to help convince the Australian public of the important role that doctors play in tobacco control may also be appropriate in future. In a survey conducted in the early 1990s, 52% of people still believed that 'a lot of doctors smoke'.[14] Despite these potential caveats, smoking rates among Australian doctors remain low, with one of the more recent surveys of hospital personnel[15] reporting that staff in the 'medical' job category had the lowest smoking rate of all (around 2%). Furthermore, smoking rates in the Australian population in general have subsequently declined, and at least part of the credit for this achievement should be given to doctors.

Table 5.1        Smoking rates among Australian doctors

| Location [a] | Smoking rate [b] | Sample size | Response rate [c] | Authors |
|---|---|---|---|---|
| **Single states** | | | | |
| Vic. | 14% | 275 | 80% | Dodds *et al.*, 1979[5] |
| **Multiple states** | | | | |
| NSW, Qld., Vic., SA | 6% | 1361 | 55% | Roche *et al.*, 1995[4] |
| NSW, Qld., Vic., SA | 4% | 908 | 55% | Roche *et al.*, 1996[8] |
| **National surveys** | | | | |
| Nationwide | 27% | 4348 | 33% | Anonymous, 1964[1] |
| Nationwide | 21% | 5708 | 40% | Anonymous, 1970[11] |
| Nationwide | 14% | 1276 | 69% | Rankin *et al.*, 1975[7] |
| Nationwide | 3% | 855 | 67% | Young & Ward, 1997[9] |
| Nationwide | 4% | 318 | 59% | McCall *et al.*, 1999[6] |

| Location [a] | Smoking rate [b] | Sample size | Response rate [c] | Authors |
|---|---|---|---|---|
| Nationwide | 3% | 311 | 73% | Young & Ward, 2001[2] |
| **Journal-based surveys** | | | | |
| Nationwide | 11% | 1500 | – | Anonymous, 1983[10] |
| Nationwide | 6% | 185 | 14% | Nyman, 1991[3] |

[a] State in which the study was undertaken (NSW=New South Wales, Qld.=Queensland, Vic.=Victoria, SA=South Australia), [b] Smoking rates rounded to the nearest whole number, [c] Response rates rounded to the nearest whole number

## 5.2    Smoking rates among American doctors

More than 50 studies have investigated tobacco-smoking habits among American doctors, as shown in Table 5.2. Most investigations were conducted as postal surveys, although one was 'distributed' to doctors at a university health sciences centre,[16] while another 'polled' members at county medical meetings.[17] At least eight studies that were predominantly conducted as postal surveys also used other methods, mainly telephone calls, to contact non-responders. Three studies were conducted across multiple states, with a fourth investigation following the same group of doctors from four different states over a 20-year period. Sample sizes ranged from under 50[18] to over 50,000 doctors,[19] with studies conducted by state medical associations generally having the largest sample sizes. Overall response rates ranged from 40% to 90% among surveys conducted in a single state, however, for the majority of multiple state and national investigations, a response rate was not listed.

Much can be learned from the studies of smoking conducted among American doctors. Some of the earliest research was a longitudinal study of 'mood-altering drugs', including tobacco, conducted between the 1930s and the 1960s.[18] By the 1960s, research into smoking among doctors was becoming more common, with at least 27 investigations being conducted in the US. Investigations conducted among multiple groups of doctors suggest that the smoking rates declined from around 40% in the 1960s to less than 10% by the 1980s. A longitudinal study of one particular group of doctors over 20 years[18] revealed a major decline in cigarette smoking, with the rate falling from 64% to 30%. Multiple studies in the same geographical location have also demonstrated similar results. In Rhode Island, where multiple smoking surveys have been conducted over an extended period, medicine had become an almost smoke-free profession by the early 1990s.[20]

Some studies examined smoking prevalence data by medical speciality. In Massachusetts during 1954, for example,[21] the lowest smoking rate was demonstrated among doctors practising in the field of preventive medicine or public health, whereas the highest rate was in proctology. In 1964,[22] it was reported that the smoking rate among Florida doctors was 40% in urology, and 37% in obstetrics/gynaecology, psychiatry and general practice.

A study conducted in 1967[23] revealed that 31% of interns and 29% of general practitioners smoked. Other early studies[24, 25] revealed that 36% of paediatricians and 42% of psychiatrists smoked cigarettes in 1968. In 1972,[26] it was reported that the smoking prevalence among Florida obstetricians / gynaecologists was 26%, whereas in general practice it was 20%. Interestingly, a study of smoking among pulmonary physicians reported that between 5% and 19% were smokers, with smoking being more common among non-practising specialists than practising specialists.[27, 28] A 1973 study of Rhode Island doctors on the other hand,[29] reported no smokers at all within that particular specialty. An investigation of cardiology conference delegates in 1984[30] reported that only 7% were cigarette smokers. Although the most frequent research on tobacco smoking rates appears to have been conducted in Rhode Island,[31–36] tobacco use among the study participants when considered by medical specialty, was far from uniform. A doctor's spouse may be an important influence on whether he or she smokes, and as such, a doctor's smoking habit probably reflects that of their partner due to assortative mating.[37] A 1968 study from New York, for example,[38] revealed that doctors who had never smoked tended to be married to non-smokers, and vice versa.

Overall, this chapter suggests that not only do very few Australian and American doctors now smoke, especially when compared to the prevalence of smoking among doctors internationally; but also, that an active professional community can make a significant difference to the lifestyle choices of its members. Much can be learned from this pivotal era of public health, where the importance of scientific knowledge, professional leadership and social responsibility helped set positive examples in the fight against tobacco use.

Table 5.2        Smoking rates among American doctors

| Location [a] | Smoking rate [b] | Sample size | Response rate [c] | Authors [d] |
|---|---|---|---|---|
| **Single states** | | | | |
| California | 21% | 2921 | 67% | CMA, 1968[39] |
| California | 15% | 151 | 76% | Wells *et al.*, 1984[40] |
| California | 8% | 221 | 62% | Fortmann *et al.*, 1985[41] |
| California | 9% | 211 | 67% | Linn *et al.*, 1986[42] |
| Connecticut | 17% | 743 | 73% | Thomas, 1968[43] |
| Florida | 30% | 3467 | 60% | Tate & Fulghum, 1965[22] |
| Florida | 18% | 5736 | 66% | Fulghum *et al.*, 1972[26] |
| Indiana | 17% | 2760 | 71% | Levitt & DeWitt, 1970[44] |

| Location [a] | Smoking rate [b] | Sample size | Response rate [c] | Authors [d] |
|---|---|---|---|---|
| Massachusetts | 35% | 4104 | – | Snegireff & Lombard, 1954[45] |
| Massachusetts | 49% | 4171 | – | Snegireff & Lombard, 1955[21] |
| Massachusetts | 39% | 4574 | – | Snegireff & Lombard, 1959[46] |
| Massachusetts | 24% | 1080 | 77% | Monson, 1970[47] |
| Massachusetts | 14% | 289 | 70% | Wyshak *et al.*, 1980[48] |
| New York | 24% | 4260 | 81% | Greenwald *et al.*, 1971[38] |
| Ohio | 10% | 144 | 77% | Browning & Thorp, 1969[49] |
| Oregon | 24% | 1794 | 90% | Meighan & Weitman, 1965[50] |
| Oregon | 39% | 1790 | 90% | Weitman *et al.*, 1967[51] |
| Pennsylvania | 42% | 2489 | 70% | Boucot & Mausner, 1964[52] |
| Pennsylvania | 19% | 296 | 47% | Glanz *et al.*, 1982[16] |
| Rhode Island | 33% | 752 | 70% | Murphy & Tierney, 1963[36] |
| Rhode Island | 23% | 1026 | 87% | Burgess & Tierney, 1969[34] |
| Rhode Island | 23% | 1026 | 87% | Burgess & Tierney, 1970[35] |
| Rhode Island | 19% | 1234 | 89% | Burgess *et al.*, 1978[32] |
| Rhode Island | 13% | 1399 | 84% | Burgess *et al.*, 1980[33] |
| Rhode Island | 8% | 1837 | 82% | Buechner *et al.*, 1986[31] |
| Wisconsin | 39% | 652 | 40% | Samp, 1963[17] |
| **Multiple states** | | | | |
| ML, MS, NY, PN | 30–64% | 45 | – | Vaillant *et al.*, 1970[18, 53] |
| CA, NB, NY | 21% | 1314 | 47–53% | Lipp & Benson, 1972[54] |

| Location [a] | Smoking rate [b] | Sample size | Response rate [c] | Authors [d] |
|---|---|---|---|---|
| AL, CA, IL, NY, PN | 11% | 61 | – | Covey & Wynder, 1981[55] |
| CA, DL, GE, PN, RI, WI | 13% | 494 | – | ACS, 1981[56] |
| **National surveys** | | | | |
| Nationwide | 29% | 4912 | 38% | NCSH, 1968[57] |
| Nationwide | 31% | 1591 | – | Coe & Brehm, 1971[23] |
| Nationwide | 36% | 287 | 38% | Eisinger, 1972[24] |
| Nationwide | 42% | 309 | 38% | Tamerin & Eisinger, 1972[25] |
| Nationwide | 48–60% | 6938 | 59% | Bruce et al., 1974[58] |
| Nationwide | 16% | 141 | – | Sterling & Weinkam, 1976[59] |
| Nationwide | 21% | ~5000 | – | MMWR, 1977[60] |
| Nationwide | 12% | 1035 | 91% | CA:ACJC, 1985[61] |
| Nationwide | 15–21% | 872,061 | – | Stellman et al., 1988[62] |
| Nationwide | 17% | 65 | – | Brackbill et al., 1988[63] |
| Nationwide | 19% | 137 | – | Nelson et al., 1994[64] |
| **Journal-based surveys** | | | | |
| Nationwide | 23% | 56,004 | – | *Modern Medicine*, 1964[19] |
| Nationwide | 38% | 1440 | – | *Medical Tribune*, 1965[65] |
| Nationwide | 23% | 2178 | – | *Modern Medicine*, 1966[66] |
| Nationwide | 27% | 562 | 56% | *Patient Care*, 1976[67] |

| Location [a] | Smoking rate [b] | Sample size | Response rate [c] | Authors [d] |
|---|---|---|---|---|
| **Unspecified locations** | | | | |
| Not specified | 16% | 262 | – | McIlreath & Cohen, 1966[68] |
| Not specified | 36% | 81 | – | Westling-Wikstrand, 1970[69] |
| Not specified | 5–19% | 594 | 27% | Sachs, 1983[27] |
| Not specified | 7% | 500 | – | Marwick, 1984[30] |

[a] State in which the study was undertaken (AL=Alabama, CA=California, DL=Delaware, IL=Illinois, ML=Maryland, MS=Massachusetts, NB=Nebraska, NY=New York, PN=Pennsylvania, RI=Rhode Island, WI=Wisconsin), [b] Smoking rates rounded to the nearest whole number, [c] Response rates rounded to the nearest whole number, [d] Author(s) of study (ACS=American Cancer Society, CA:ACJC=CA: A Cancer Journal for Clinicians, CMA=California Medical Association, MMWR=Morbidity and Mortality Weekly Report, NCSH=National Clearinghouse for Smoking and Health)

# Chapter 6

# Discussion and conclusions

*This chapter provides a concluding discussion on the topic of smoking among healthcare workers. Overall, it is clear that much can be learned from an examination of smoking trends within the healthcare workforce and students. While there are certainly common issues faced by healthcare workforces around the world, significant cultural and social influences also exist, making it difficult to adopt a 'one-size-fits-all' solution. Tobacco control among current and future healthcare professionals will clearly need a multifaceted approach to confront the high smoking rates that are still being reported among this group in various countries.*

## 6.1    Discussion

This book provides a comprehensive examination of tobacco usage within the healthcare profession internationally. Aside from the range of smoking rates identified by subdiscipline, country and year, our book has also revealed a number of other key findings. Firstly, at its broadest level, it would appear that the literature on tobacco-smoking among the healthcare profession is rapidly increasing. It is difficult to confirm whether this increase actually indicates that more research is being conducted, or simply that a greater proportion of research is now being listed on databases and detected with search engines. At the same time, there is the possibility of a bias in the publication of biomedical research, caused by the fact that countries with lower socioeconomic rankings tend to publish less research in international journals.[1]

Another issue encountered when examining smoking research was that of survey response rates. Low response rates are particularly important in surveys where the measured outcome may be socially undesirable, as participants may be reluctant to make certain admissions, or even return their survey at all. Healthcare professionals who smoke tobacco may feel guilty about their habit for example, and as a result, may underreport it.[2] This phenomenon is not new, however, with the issue of responder bias having been recognised as a methodological limitation of survey-based research for many years. In 1970, for example, an examination of smoking habits among doctors in the US[3] found that although 90% of all non-smokers responded to an initial mailed survey, only 77% of smokers had done so. Later analysis of the smoking prevalence among survey respondents when compared to non-respondents also revealed wide discrepancies (with smoking rates of 23% among respondents versus 46% among non-respondents). Similarly, a postal survey of US nurses revealed that the smoking rate among those who responded to their initial mailing (26%) was lower than among those who responded to a second follow-up mailing (30%).[4] Furthermore, a survey of Japanese doctors revealed that the prevalence of smoking among those who responded to the second, third and fourth mailings was approximately 1.5 times higher than for those who had replied to the initial mailing.[5] These results suggest that healthcare professionals who consume tobacco may be reluctant to complete and return smoking-related questionnaires. It is imperative therefore that healthcare researchers carefully consider these issues when designing their investigations.

Another issue to consider when examining published research on this topic relates to the definition of a 'smoker', along with a general lack of consensus regarding what tobacco product the respondent actually smoked. Although most authors referred to their subjects as either current smokers or non-smokers, the type of tobacco they smoked was classified in many different categories such as cigarettes only, pipes only, cigars only, pipes and cigars, pipes or cigars, cigarettes or pipes or cigars, and so on. Regarding the time scale, some studies had used smoking recall periods ranging from one week to one month in their definition of the term 'smoker'. This lack of standardisation in tobacco smoking research has previously been noted among studies conducted with healthcare professionals, and probably arises due to the inherent difficulties in assessing smoking habits over time, and the fact that most investigations simply report the prevalence of smoking within the surveyed group. Aside from absolute smoking rates, an examination of the published literature also suggests that the relative epidemiological quality of research investigations has fluctuated over time, making it difficult to directly compare the results from one individual study to another.

Healthcare professionals have always had an important responsibility to convince their patients not to smoke, as they are generally viewed as exemplars by the community, and also serve as providers of support, information and encouragement in helping patients to achieve such a goal. Our review of published smoking studies that had been conducted among doctors revealed that their smoking habits certainly vary from region to region, and that they are not uniformly low when viewed from an international perspective. Comparison with other health professionals suggests that doctors probably smoke less than nurses in the same location, but not as infrequently as dentists. An overall low rate of tobacco usage in the dental profession suggests that they smoke at one of the lowest rates among all health professionals, and much lower than that of the communities in which they live. There were some notable exceptions however, namely in Brazil,[6] Jordan[7] and Italy,[8] where around one-third of the dentists surveyed were smokers. While nurses' tobacco usage has decreased in many countries during recent years, the trend is far from uniform internationally, and some developed nations still appear to have high smoking rates among their nursing staff. Moreover, the prevalence and distribution of tobacco use has been shown to vary widely depending on the time period when the study was undertaken and also the nursing discipline which was sampled.

Encouraging healthcare professionals who smoke to quit their habit remains a contentious issue for tobacco control. For example, the *British Doctor's Study* revealed that quitting smoking at any age is clearly effective at reducing the loss of life expectancy due to smoking.[9] However, as this review has shown, the US medical profession was still not entirely smoke free by 1984, even though doctors were known to have given up smoking at a higher rate than any other professional group.[10] Targeting medical students may represent one way forward in this regard, although smoking habits that begin in medical school may be particularly difficult to address. A study of Malaysian doctors, for example,[11] found that around half were already smoking before they even entered medical school. Additionally, some of the earliest US studies[12, 13] revealed that a large proportion of US medical students were using tobacco products on entry to medical school. Recent research suggests, however, that US medical students now have some of the lowest rates of smoking in the world,[14] similar to their dental student counterparts.[15]

From a broader perspective, it is also important to consider whether the issue of tobacco smoking in the healthcare industry should be interpreted as a simple problem in itself, or as 'a signpost to more fundamental issues within the profession'.[16] Even if the results from smoking interventions appear to be a little disappointing, it is important to remember that the value of anti-smoking interventions themselves should never be underestimated. Preventing healthcare professionals commencing smoking, as well as helping those who already smoke to quit, represents a critical issue for future tobacco control research. In meeting these needs, it has been found that health promotion coordinators and peer support groups may be useful.[17] It has also been suggested that health promotion skills could be integrated into contemporary education.[18]

When considering the issue of tobacco smoking among health professionals, it is important to recognise future directions for research in this field. While the findings of this book clearly suggest that many health professionals still smoke tobacco, it is important to view the results from a wider perspective of health. Aside from encouraging young health professionals, particularly students, not to smoke, future health policies should also aim to strengthen their resolve to quit.[19] Health professionals know well the dangers that tobacco use poses them, and at least 20 years ago, it had been noted that many who did smoke certainly felt guilty about their habit.[2] As such, the prevention of smoking itself and the promotion of tobacco cessation activities remain important goals in both practice and research. Despite this fact, relatively few studies have reported the results of smoking intervention studies, and few of those interventions that have been conducted could be described as being totally successful.

Aside from intervention studies, an individual smoker's attitude towards quitting has also been shown to be important. In a US study, for example, a competition was held to help nurses quit smoking.[20] At the end of the two-week intervention period, however, not one nurse even attended the program session. While the authors subsequently referred to their trial as a 'failed experiment',[20] they were able to identify some potential reasons as to why this situation may have occurred. Some head nurses, for example, had apparently surmised that any staff who wanted to use the quit smoking program would have already done so, while further harassment of the remaining hard-core smokers was deemed to be inappropriate.[20] It is this potentially 'unreachable' group of dedicated smokers that would seem to be a key area in need of attention, with regard to future smoking and tobacco control research within the healthcare profession.

From a global perspective, the World Health Organization's (WHO) Tobacco Free Initiative[21] has proposed general strategies for promoting tobacco control, particularly in its publications on tobacco smoking among the world's younger population.[22] While many of these strategies are applicable for future use among healthcare students, some progress is already being made. A ten-year follow-up study of European dental schools, for example, found that almost three quarters of European dental schools now taught students anti-smoking (or 'quit' smoking) advice and expected them to give such advice to patients.[23] A contemporary survey of dental professionals in the UK also revealed that 90% of dental practices were now smoke-free environments.[24]

## 6.2    Conclusions

Overall, the examination of tobacco smoking research covered in this book has revealed some interesting findings. Firstly, the absolute rate of tobacco usage appears to vary by country and healthcare subdiscipline. There were also differences between the smoking rates of healthcare professionals and their student counterparts. Among student cohorts, many cross-sectional investigations suggest that the prevalence of smoking may increase as one passes through the more senior grades, however it is difficult to ascertain whether this trend directly reflects university seniority, increasing age or both. Regardless of the reason, there can be no doubt that education represents a critical issue in smoking cessation for both medical students and the general public alike. Similarly, while the results from some intervention studies appear to be a little disappointing, the value of anti-smoking interventions for healthcare students should not be underestimated. Preventing the next generation of healthcare worker from commencing smoking and helping those who already smoke to give up their habit represents a critical issue for educators. It is only when healthcare becomes a truly smoke-free profession that healthcare professionals can claim to be exemplars of the highest order.

# Appendices

## Appendix 1

## Smoking rates among veterinarians

More than 10 published studies were located and examined for this Appendix, as shown in Appendix Table 1. Response rates for smoking studies conducted among veterinarians have ranged from 23% to 86%, although many achieved a greater than 50% response. One of the earliest investigations to document smoking rates among this group appears to have been conducted in the US during 1986, where it was reported that 5% of female veterinary school graduates currently smoked.[1] Five years later, a study of respiratory diseases from the Southern Netherlands documented a much higher smoking rate of 29%. A further 34% of the Dutch veterinarians were ex-smokers.[2] Two statewide studies from the US were conducted in the mid-1990s, one in Minnesota[3] and another in California,[4] which revealed similar smoking rates of between 6% and 7%. The lowest smoking rate appears to be 2% reported by participants at an American Swine Veterinarians' conference during 2002.[5] In the same year, a study of Michigan veterinarians documented a smoking rate of 5%.[6] The highest international smoking rate in the veterinary profession appears to be in Germany, where 19% of those surveyed were current smokers and 26% ex-smokers.[7]

Three studies have investigated tobacco smoking rates among Australian veterinarians, with the first being a national survey of graduates from four Australian veterinary schools between 1960 and 2000. Although it predominantly focussed on workplace injuries, a non-smoking rate of 73% and an ex-smoking rate of 22% were reported.[8] In 2007, an article was published which analysed data from this same study,[9] reporting that among female veterinarians, current smoking rates were 5%, with 13% ex-smokers and 81% having never smoked. Indeed, tobacco usage rates among Australian veterinarians were so low in the 2004–05 *National Health Survey*, that this job category did not appear in detailed analysis of tobacco smoking rates by occupation.[10] A third study of smoking habits among veterinarians in Queensland, Australia, was published in 2010 and reported a prevalence of 3%.[11]

Appendix Table 1    Smoking rates among veterinarians

| | Smoking rate [a] | | | Study details | | |
| Country | All | Male | Female | Sample size | Response rate [b] | Authors |
| --- | --- | --- | --- | --- | --- | --- |
| Australia | 5% | – | – | 2800 | 48% | Fritschi *et al.*, 2006[8] |
| Australia | – | – | 5% | 1197 | 43% | Shirangi *et al.*, 2007[9] |
| Australia | 3% | 3% | 3% | 567 | 55% | Smith *et al.*, 2010[11] |
| Germany | 19% | – | – | 1060 | 53% | Harling *et al.*, 2009[7] |
| Netherlands | 29% | – | – | 497 | 73% | Tielen *et al.*, 1996[2] |
| United States | – | – | 5% | 462 | 86% | Schenker *et al.*, 1990[1] |
| United States | 6% | – | – | 688 | 67–69% | Gabel & Gerberich, 2002[3] |
| United States | 7% | 9% | 5% | 1353 | 73% | Susitaival *et al.*, 2003[4] |
| United States | 2% | – | – | 122 | 23% | Andersen *et al.*, 2004[5] |
| United States | 2% | – | – | 58 | 7% | Poole *et al.*, 2007[12] |
| United States | 5% | – | – | 175 | 71% | Wilkins *et al.*, 2009[6] |

[a] Smoking rates rounded to the nearest whole number, [b] Response rates rounded to the nearest whole number

## Appendix 2

### Smoking rates among veterinary students

Despite an extensive literature search undertaken for this Appendix, only two studies (describing three student groups) appear to have been published which document the smoking rate of veterinary students, as shown in Appendix Table 2. The first, an investigation of students in the United Kingdom (UK) reported a smoking rate of 5% for female and 28% for male students.[13] A more recent study, this time conducted at two veterinary schools in the US, documented a smoking rate of between 9% and 15%, although prevalence rates were not reported by gender at either location.

Appendix Table 2    Smoking rates among veterinary students

| | Smoking Rate [a] | | | Study Details | | |
| Country | All | Male | Female | Sample Size | Response Rate [b] | Authors |
|---|---|---|---|---|---|---|
| United Kingdom | – | 28% | 5% | 123 | 100% | Webb *et al.*, 1997[13] |
| United States | 9% | – | – | 231 | 80% | Hofmeister *et al.*, 2010[14] |
| United States | 15% | – | – | 250 | 62% | Hofmeister *et al.*, 2010[14] |

[a] Smoking rates rounded to the nearest whole number, [b] Response rates rounded to the nearest whole number

## Appendix 3

## Prior publications related to this book

Parts of this book are based on some earlier scientific articles written by the authors and used with kind permission of the Editors and publishers: BioMed Central, Elsevier, FDI World Dental Press Ltd, MedKnow Publications, SAGE Publications and the Wiley Company. The full reference for each article is listed below, along with a web link to the definitive version, correct as of 2011.

### Chapter 1

Smith DR. Tobacco control and the nursing profession. *Nursing & Health Sciences* 2010; **12**: 1–3 (onlinelibrary.wiley.com/doi/10.111/j.1442-2018.2010.0058.x/full).

### Chapter 3

Smith DR, Leggat PA. An international review of tobacco smoking in the medical profession: 1974–2004. *BMC Public Health* 2007; 7: 115 (www.biomedcentral.com/1471-2458/7/115).

Smith DR, Leggat PA. A comparison of tobacco smoking among dentists in 15 countries. *International Dental Journal* 2006; **56**: 283–88 (onlinelibrary.wiley.com/doi/10.1111/j.1875-595X.2006.tb00102.x/abstract).

Smith DR, Leggat PA. An international review of tobacco smoking research in the nursing profession, 1976–2006. *Journal of Research in Nursing* 2007; **12**: 165–81 (jrn.sagepub.com/content/12/2/165.abstract).

### Chapter 4

Smith DR, Leggat PA. An international review of tobacco smoking among medical students. *Journal of Postgraduate Medicine* 2007; **53**: 55–62 (www.jpgmonline.com/article.asp?issn=0022-3859;year=2007;volume=53;issue=1;spage=55;epage=62;aulast=smith;type=0).

Smith DR, Leggat PA. An international review of tobacco smoking among dental students in 19 countries. *International Dental Journal* 2007; **57**: 452–58 (onlinelibrary.wiley.com/doi/10.1111/j.1875-595X.2007.tb00149.x/abstract).

Smith DR. A systematic review of tobacco smoking among nursing students. *Nurse Education in Practice* 2007; **7**: 293–302 (www.sciencedirect.com/science/article/pii/S1471595306001004).

*Chapter 5*

Smith DR, Leggat PA. The historical decline of tobacco smoking among Australian physicians: 1964–1997. *Tobacco Induced Diseases* 2008; **4**: 13 (Epub: www.tobaccoinduceddiseases.com/content/4/1/13).

Smith DR. The historical decline of tobacco smoking among United States physicians: 1949–1984. *Tobacco Induced Diseases* 2008; **4**: 9 (Epub: www.tobaccoinduceddiseases.com/content/4/1/9).

*Chapter 6*

Smith DR. Tobacco control and the nursing profession. *Nursing & Health Sciences* 2010; 12: 1–3 (onlinelibrary.wiley.com/doi/10.1111/j.1442-2018.2010.00518.x/full).

*Appendices*

Smith DR, Leggat PA, Speare,R. The latest endangered species in Australia: a tobacco-smoking veterinarian. *Australian Veterinary Journal* 2010; **88**: 369–70 (onlinelibrary.wiley.com/doi/10.1111/j.1751-0813.2010.00614.x/abstract).

# About the authors

## Derek R. Smith

Derek R. Smith is Professor of Environmental and Occupational Health and Deputy Director (Research) at the Central Coast Campus of the University of Newcastle in New South Wales, Australia. He is active in many different research areas including environmental and occupational health, public health, epidemiology, bibliometrics and medical history. He has published over 200 scientific articles and presented at numerous domestic and international conferences.

## Peter A. Leggat

Peter A. Leggat is Professor and Deputy Head at the School of Public Health, Tropical Medicine and Rehabilitation Sciences, and Associate Dean for Faculty Affairs, Faculty of Medicine, Health and Molecular Sciences at James Cook University in Townsville, Australia. He is a specialist in public health medicine and is a certified Medical Review Officer. He has published over 450 journal articles, 50 chapters and 20 monographs, and presented more than 300 papers at national and international meetings.

# References

## Chapter 1


1. Wipfli H, Samet JM. Global economic and health benefits of tobacco control: part 1. *Clin Pharmacol Ther* 2009; **86:** 263–71.

2. Smith DR, Leggat PA. Tobacco smoking by occupation in Australia: results from the 2004 to 2005 National Health Survey. *J Occup Environ Med* 2007; **49:** 437–45.

3. Garfinkel L. Trends in cigarette smoking in the United States. *Prev Med* 1997; **26:** 447–50.

4. Giovino GA. Epidemiology of tobacco use in the United States. *Oncogene* 2002; **21:** 7326–40.

5. Brill AA. Tobacco and the individual. *Int J Psychoanal* 1922; **3:** 430–44.

6. When "more doctors smoked Camels": cigarette advertising in the journal. *NY State J Med* 1983; **83:** 1347–52.

7. Kawane H. When doctors advertised cigarettes. *Tob Control* 1993; **2:** 45.

8. Hammond EC, Horn D. The relationship between human smoking habits and death rates: a follow-up study of 187,766 men. *J Am Med Assoc* 1954; **155:** 1316–28.

9. Hammond EC, Horn D. Smoking and death rates: report on forty-four months of follow-up of 187,783 men. 2. Death rates by cause. *J Am Med Assoc* 1958; **166:** 1294–308.

10. Hammond EC, Horn D. Smoking and death rates; report on forty-four months of follow-up of 187,783 men. I. Total mortality. *J Am Med Assoc* 1958; **166:** 1159–72.

11. Mahaney FX, Jr. Oldtime ads tout health benefits of smoking: tobacco industry had doctors' help. *J Natl Cancer Inst* 1994; **86:** 1048–49.

12. Gardner MN, Brandt AM. "The doctors' choice is America's choice": the physician in US cigarette advertisements, 1930–1953. *Am J Public Health* 2006; **96:** 222–32.

13. Garland LH. The smoking physician. *CA Cancer J Clin* 1959; **9:** 60–61.

14. Smoking and Health. Report of the advisory committee to the surgeon general of the public health service. Washington: U.S. Department of Health, Education and Welfare, 1964.

15. Hammond EC, Van Griethuysen TH, Dibeler JB, Sneddon AM, Halligan W. Smoking habits and disease in New York State. *N Y State J Med* 1965; **65:** 2557–61.

16. Froelicher ES, Kohlman VC. Tobacco free nurses. The facts on nurses and smoking. *J Cardiopulm Rehabil* 2005; **25**: 198–99.

17. Adriaanse H, van Reek J. Physicians' smoking and its exemplary effect. *Scand J Prim Health Care* 1989; **7**: 193–96.

18. Smoking and health: A physician's responsibility. A statement of the joint committee on smoking and health. American College of Chest Physicians, American Thoracic Society, Asia Pacific Society of Respirology, Canadian Thoracic Society, European Respiratory Society, International Union Against Tuberculosis and Lung Disease. *Eur Respir J* 1995; **8**: 1808–11.

19. Chapman S. Doctors who smoke. *Br Med J* 1995; **311**: 142–43.

20. Centers for Disease Control and Prevention (CDC). Smoking control among health-care workers – World No-Tobacco Day, 1993. *MMWR Morb Mortal Wkly Rep* 1993; **42**: 365–67.

21. Garfinkel L. Cigarette smoking among physicians and other health professionals, 1959–1972. *CA Cancer J Clin* 1976; **26**: 373–75.

22. Sachs DP. Smoking habits of pulmonary physicians. *N Engl J Med* 1983; **309**: 799.

## Chapter 2


1. Melby CS. Examining the future of professional journals. *Nurs Health Sci* 2005; **7**: 219–20.

2. Rahman M, Fukui T. Biomedical publication – global profile and trend. *Public Health* 2003; **117**: 274–80.

3. United States National Library of Medicine (NLM) Webpage: International Committee of Medical Journal Editors (ICMJE) uniform requirements for manuscripts submitted to biomedical journals: sample references. Available online at: www.nlm.nih.gov/bsd/uniform_requirements.html (Accessed: 27 May 2011)

4. Patrick DL, Cheadle A, Thompson DC, Diehr P, Koepsell T, Kinne S. The validity of self-reported smoking: a review and meta-analysis. *Am J Public Health* 1994; **84**: 1086–93.

5. Vartiainen E, Seppala T, Lillsunde P, Puska P. Validation of self-reported smoking by serum cotinine measurement in a community-based study. *J Epidemiol Community Health* 2002; **56**: 167–70.

6. Soto Mas FG, Papenfuss RL, Jacobson HE, Hsu CE, Urrutia-Rojas X, Kane WM. Hispanic physicians' tobacco intervention practices: A cross-sectional survey study. *BMC Public Health* 2005; **5**: 120.

7. Doll R, Peto R, Wheatley K, Gray R, Sutherland I. Mortality in relation to smoking: 40 years' observations on male British doctors. *Br Med J* 1994; **309**: 901–11.

8. Fowler G, Mant D, Fuller A, Jones L. The "Help Your Patient Stop" initiative. Evaluation of smoking prevalence and dissemination of WHO/UICC guidelines in UK general practice. *Lancet* 1989; **1**: 1253–55.

## Chapter 3


1. Uysal MA, Dilmen N, Karasulu L, Demir T. Smoking habits among physicians in Istanbul and their attitudes regarding anti-smoking legislation. *Tuberk Toraks* 2007; **55**: 350–55.

2. Jiang Y, Ong MK, Tong EK, Yang Y, Nan Y, Gan Q, Hu TW. Chinese physicians and their smoking knowledge, attitudes, and practices. *Am J Prev Med* 2007; **33**: 15–22.

3. Yaacob I, Abdullah ZA. Smoking habits and attitudes among doctors in a Malaysian hospital. *Southeast Asian J Trop Med Public Health* 1993; **24**: 28–31.

4. Soto Mas FG, Papenfuss RL, Jacobson HE, Hsu CE, Urrutia-Rojas X, Kane WM. Hispanic physicians' tobacco intervention practices: A cross-sectional survey study. *BMC Public Health* 2005; **5**: 120.

5. Doll R, Peto R, Wheatley K, Gray R, Sutherland I. Mortality in relation to smoking: 40 years' observations on male British doctors. *Br Med J* 1994; **309**: 901–11.

6. Frank E. The Women Physicians' Health Study: Background, objectives, and methods. *J Am Med Womens Assoc* 1995; **50**: 64–66.

7. Frank E, Lutz LJ. Characteristics of women US family physicians. *Arch Fam Med* 1999; **8**: 313–18.

8. Frank E, Rothenberg R, Lewis C, Belodoff BF. Correlates of physicians' prevention-related practices. Findings from the Women Physicians' Health Study. *Arch Fam Med* 2000; **9**: 359–67.

9. Hay DR. Cigarette smoking by New Zealand doctors: Results from the 1976 population census. *NZ Med J* 1980; **91**: 285–88.

10. Hay DR. Intercensal trends in cigarette smoking by New Zealand doctors and nurses. *NZ MedJ*1984; **97**: 253–55.

11. Hay DR. Cigarette smoking by New Zealand doctors and nurses: Results from the 1996 population census. *NZ Med J* 1998; **111**: 102–04.

12. Roche AM, Parle MD, Saunders JB. Managing alcohol and drug problems in general practice: A survey of trainees' knowledge, attitudes and educational requirements. *Aust NZ J Public Health* 1996; **20**: 401–08.

13. Roche AM, Parle MD, Stubbs JM, Hall W, Saunders JB. Management and treatment efficacy of drug and alcohol problems: What do doctors believe? *Addiction* 1995; **90**: 1357–66.

14. Young JM, Ward JE. Declining rates of smoking among medical practitioners. *Med J Aust* 1997; **167**: 232.

15. Edwards R, Bowler T, Atkinson J, Wilson N. Low and declining cigarette smoking rates among doctors and nurses: 2006 New Zealand Census data. *NZ Med J* 2008; **121**: 43–51.

16. Ponniah S, Bloomfield A. An update on tobacco smoking among New Zealand health care workers, the current picture, 2006. *NZ Med J* 2008; **121**: 103–05.

17. Doll R, Peto R, Boreham J, Sutherland I. Mortality in relation to smoking: 50 years' observations on male British doctors. *Br Med J* 2004; **328**: 1519–28.

18. Doll R, Peto R, Boreham J, Sutherland I. Mortality from cancer in relation to smoking: 50 years' observations on British doctors. *Br J Cancer* 2005; **92**: 426–29.

19. Josseran L, King G, Guilbert P, Davis J, Brucker G. Smoking by French general practitioners: Behaviour, attitudes and practice. *Eur J Public Health* 2005; **15**: 33–38.

20. Josseran L, King G, Velter A, Dressen C, Grizeau D. Smoking behavior and opinions of French general practitioners. *J Natl Med Assoc* 2000; **92**: 382–90.

21. Tessier JF, Rene L, Nejjari C, Belougne D, Moulin J, Freour P. Attitudes and opinions of French general practitioners towards tobacco. *Tob Control* 1993; **2**: 226–30.

22. La Vecchia C, Scarpino V, Malvezzi I, Baldi G. A survey of smoking among Italian doctors. *J Epidemiol Community Health* 2000; **54**: 320.

23. Nardini S, Bertoletti R, Rastelli V, Donner CF. The influence of personal tobacco smoking on the clinical practice of Italian chest physicians. *Eur Respir J* 1998; **12**: 1450–53.

24. Nardini S, Bertoletti R, Rastelli V, Ravelli L, Donner CF. Personal smoking habit and attitude toward smoking among the health staff of a general hospital. *Monaldi Arch Chest Dis* 1998; **53**: 74–78.

25. Pizzo AM, Chellini E, Grazzini G, Cardone A, Badellino F. Italian general practitioners and smoking cessation strategies. *Tumori* 2003; **89**: 250–54.

26. Zanetti F, Gambi A, Bergamaschi A, Gentilini F, De Luca G, Monti C. Smoking habits, exposure to passive smoking and attitudes to a non-smoking policy among hospital staff. *Public Health* 1998; **112**: 57–62.

27. Kaetsu A, Fukushima T, Moriyama M, Shigematsu T. Change of the smoking behavior and related lifestyle variables among physicians in Fukuoka, Japan: A longitudinal study. *J Epidemiol* 2002; **12**: 208–16.

28. Kaetsu A, Fukushima T, Moriyama M, Shigematsu T. Smoking behavior and related lifestyle variables among physicians in Fukuoka, Japan: A cross-sectional study. *J Epidemiol* 2002; **12**: 199–207.

29. Kawane H. Smoking among older chest physicians. *Chest* 1991; **99**: 526.

30. Kawane H. The prevalence of smoking among physicians in Japan. *Am J Public Health* 1993; **83**: 1640.

31. Kawane H. Smoking among Japanese physicians. *JAMA* 2001; **286**: 917.

32. Kawane H, Soejima R. Smoking among doctors in a medical school hospital. *Kawasaki Med J* 1996; **22**: 211–16.

33. Ohida T, Sakurai H, Mochizuki Y, Kamal AM, Takemura S, Minowa M. Smoking prevalence and attitudes toward smoking among Japanese physicians. *JAMA* 2001; **285**: 2643–48.

34. Kaneita Y, Sakurai H, Tsuchiya T, Ohida T. Changes in smoking prevalence and attitudes to smoking among Japanese physicians between 2000 and 2004. *Public Health* 2008; **122:** 882–90.

35. Kawahara K, Ohida T, Osaki Y, Mochizuki Y, Minowa M, Yamaguchi N. Study of the smoking behavior of medical doctors in Fukui, Japan and their antismoking measures. *J Epidemiol* 2000; **10:** 157–62.

36. Kawakami M, Nakamura S, Fumimoto H, Takizawa J, Baba M. Relation between smoking status of physicians and their enthusiasm to offer smoking cessation advice. *Intern Med* 1997; **36:** 162–65.

37. Hodgetts G, Broers T, Godwin M. Smoking behaviour, knowledge and attitudes among family medicine physicians and nurses in Bosnia and Herzegovina. *BMC Fam Pract* 2004; **5:** 12.

38. Parna K, Rahu K, Barengo NC, Rahu M, Sandstrom PH, Jormanainen VJ. Comparison of knowledge, attitudes and behaviour regarding smoking among Estonian and Finnish physicians. *Soz Praventivmed* 2005; **50:** 378–88.

39. Parna K, Rahu K, Rahu M. Smoking habits and attitudes towards smoking among Estonian physicians. *Public Health* 2005; **119:** 390–99.

40. Gunes G, Karaoglu L, Genc MF, Pehlivan E, Egri M. University hospital physicians' attitudes and practices for smoking cessation counseling in Malatya, Turkey. *Patient Educ Couns* 2005; **56:** 147–53.

41. An DTM, Huy NV, Phong DN. Smoking among Vietnamese health professionals: Knowledge, beliefs, attitudes, and health care practice. *Asia Pac J Public Health* 2008; **20:** 7–15.

42. Nollen NL, Adewale S, Okuyemi KS, Ahluwalia JS, Parakoyi A. Workplace tobacco policies and smoking cessation practices of physicians. *J Natl Med Assoc* 2004; **96:** 838–42.

43. de Assis Viegas CA, de Andrade AP, Silvestre Rda S. Characteristics of smoking among physicians in the Federal District of Brazil. *J Bras Pneumol* 2007; **33:** 76–80.

44. An LC, Bernhardt TS, Bluhm J, Bland P, Center B, Ahluwalia JS. Treatment of tobacco use as a chronic medical condition: Primary care physicians' self-reported practice patterns. *Prev Med* 2004; **38:** 574–85.

45. Brink SG, Gottlieb NH, McLeroy KR, Wisotzky M, Burdine JN. A community view of smoking cessation counselling in the practices of physicians and dentists. *Public Health Rep* 1994; **109:** 135–42.

46. Tong EK, Strouse R, Hall J, Kovac M, Schroeder SA. National survey of U.S. health professionals' smoking prevalence, cessation practices, and beliefs. *Nicotine Tob Res* 2010; **12:** 724–33.

47. Davies PD, Rajan K. Attitudes to smoking and smoking habit among the staff of a hospital. *Thorax* 1989; **44:** 378–81.

48. Polyzos A, Gennatas C, Veslemes M, Daskalopoulou E, Stamatiadis D, Katsilambros N. The smoking-cessation promotion practices of physician smokers in Greece. *J Cancer Educ* 1995; **10:** 78–81.

49. Li HZ, Fish D, Zhou X. Increase in cigarette smoking and decline of anti-smoking counselling among Chinese physicians: 1987–1996. *Health Prom Int* 1999; **14:** 123–31.

50. Bener A, Gomes J, Anderson JAD. Smoking habits among physicians in two gulf countries. *J R Soc Health* 1993; **113:** 298–301.

51. Sarkar D, Dhand R, Malhotra A, Malhotra S, Sharma BK. Perceptions and attitude towards tobacco smoking among doctors in Chandigarh. *Indian J Chest Dis Allied Sci* 1990; **32:** 1–9.

52. Ballal SG. Cigarette smoking and respiratory symptoms among Sudanese doctors. *East Afr Med J* 1984; **61:** 95–103.

53. Kono S, Ikeda M, Tokudome S, Nishizumi M, Kuratsune M. Smoking and mortalities from cancer, coronary heart disease and stroke in male Japanese physicians. *J Cancer Res Clin Oncol* 1985; **110:** 161–64.

54. Sotiropoulos A, Gikas A, Spanou E, Dimitrelos D, Karakostas F, Skliros E, Apostolou O, Politakis P, Pappas S. Smoking habits and associated factors among Greek physicians. *Public Health* 2007; **121:** 333–40.

55. Smith DR, Wei N, Zhang YJ, Wang RS. Tobacco smoking habits among a cross-section of rural physicians in China. *Aust J Rural Health* 2006; **14:** 66–71.

56. Cheng KK, Lam TH. Smoking among young doctors in Hong Kong: A message to medical educators. *Med Educ* 1990; **24:** 158–63.

57. Nutbeam D, Catford J. Modifiable risks for cardiovascular disease among general practitioners in Wales. *Public Health* 1990; **104:** 353–61.

58. Samuels N. Smoking among hospital doctors in Israel and their attitudes regarding anti-smoking legislation. *Public Health* 1997; **111:** 285–88.

59. Scott HD, Tierney JT, Buechner JS, Waters WJ. Smoking rates among Rhode Island physicians: Achieving a smoke-free society. *Am J Prev Med* 1992; **8:** 86–90.

60. Tapia-Conyer R, Cravioto P, de la Rosa B, Galvan F, Garcia-de la Torre G, Kuri P. Cigarette smoking; knowledge and attitudes among Mexican physicians. *Salud Publica Mex* 1997; **39:** 507–12.

61. Hill HA, Braithwaite RL. Attitudes, beliefs, and practices regarding smoking and smoking cessation among African-American physicians and dentists. *J Natl Med Assoc* 1997; **89:** 745–51.

62. Kenna GA, Wood MD. The prevalence of alcohol, cigarette and illicit drug use and problems among dentists. *J Am Dent Assoc* 2005; **136:** 1023–32.

63. Wyshak G, Lamb GA, Lawrence RS, Curran WJ. A profile of the health-promoting behaviors of physicians and lawyers. *N Engl J Med* 1980; **303:** 104–07.

64. Heloma A, Reijula K, Tikkanen J, Nykyri E. The attitudes of occupational health personnel to smoking at work. *Am J Ind Med* 1998; **34:** 73–78.

65. Davis RM. When doctors smoke. *Tob Control* 1993; **2:** 187–88.

66. Christmas BW, Hay DR. The smoking habits of New Zealand doctors: A review after ten years. *NZ Med J* 1976; **83:** 391–94.

67. Dekker HM, Looman CWN, Adriaanse HP, Van Der Maas PJ. Prevalence of smoking in physicians and medical students, and the generation effect in the Netherlands. *Soc Sci Med* 1993; **36:** 817–22.

68. Jormanainen VJ, Myllykangas MT, Nissinen A. Decreasing the prevalence of smoking among Finnish physicians. *Eur J Public Health* 1997; **7:** 318–20.

69. Waalkens HJ, Cohen Schotanus J, Adriaanse H, Knol K. Smoking habits in medical students and physicians in Groningen, The Netherlands. *Eur Respir J* 1992; **5:** 49–52.

70. Hughes PH, Baldwin DC, Sheehan DV, Conard S, Storr CL. Resident physician substance use, by specialty. *Am J Psychiatry* 1992; **149:** 1348–54.

71. McEwen A, West R. Smoking cessation activities by general practitioners and practice nurses. *Tob Control* 2001; **10:** 27–32.

72. Audet B. When it comes to smoking, Japanese MDs do not set a good example for their patients. *CMAJ* 1994; **150:** 1673–74.

73. Stillman FA, Becker DM, Swank RT, Hantula D, Moses H, Glantz S. Ending smoking at the Johns Hopkins Medical Institutions. An evaluation of smoking prevalence and indoor air pollution. *JAMA* 1990; **264:** 1565–69.

74. Bartscherer DJ, Reichert VC, Folan P, DeGaetano C, Jacobsen DR, Miceli L, Kohn N, Talwar A. Tobacco and the health care industry. *Clin Occup Environ Med* 2006; **5:** 55–71, viii.

75. Seiler ER. Smoking habits of doctors and their spouses in south-east Scotland. *J R Coll Gen Pract* 1983; **33:** 598.

76. Hay DR, Christmas BW. The smoking habits of women doctors and doctors' wives in New Zealand. *Prev Med* 1976; **5:** 78–88.

77. Barengo NC, Sandstrom HP, Jormanainen VJ, Myllykangas M. Attitudes and behaviours in smoking cessation among general practitioners in Finland 2001. *Soz Praventivmed* 2005; **50:** 355–60.

78. Rankin DW, Gray NJ, Hill DJ, Evans DR. Attitudes and smoking habits of Australian doctors. *Med J Aust* 1975; **2:** 822–24.

79. Dodds AM, Rankin DW, Hill DJ, Gray NJ. Attitudes and smoking habits of doctors in Victoria. *Community Health Stud* 1979; **3:** 28–31.

80. Joossens L, Demedts M, Prignot J, Bartsch P, Gyselen A. Smoking habits of Belgian physicians: Effects of consonancy behaviour and of age. *Acta Clin Belg* 1987; **42:** 457–61.

81. Senior SL. Study of smoking habits in hospital and attitudes of medical staff towards smoking. *CMAJ* 1982; **126:** 131–33.

82. De Koninck M, Guay H, Bourbonnais R, Bergeron P. Physical, mental, and reproductive health of Quebec women physicians. *J Am Med Womens Assoc* 1995; **50:** 59–63.

83. Yan J, Xiao S, Ouyang D, Jiang D, He C, Yi S. Smoking behavior, knowledge, attitudes and practice among health care providers in Changsha City, China. *Nicotine Tob Res* 2008; **10:** 737–44.

84. Zhou J, Abdullah AS, Pun VC, Huang D, Lu S, Luo S. Smoking status and cessation counseling practices among physicians, Guangxi, China, 2007. *Prev Chronic Dis* 2010; **7:** 1–10.

85. Grossman DW, Knox JJ, Nash C, Jimenez JG. Smoking: Attitudes of Costa Rican physicians and opportunities for intervention. *Bull World Health Organ* 1999; **77:** 315–22.

86. Willaing I, Jorgensen T, Iversen L. How does individual smoking behaviour among hospital staff influence their knowledge of the health consequences of smoking? *Scand J Public Health* 2003; **31:** 149–55.

87. Kannegaard PN, Kreiner S, Gregersen P, Goldstein H. Smoking habits and attitudes to smoking 2001 among hospital staff at a Danish hospital – Comparison with a similar study 1999. *Prev Med* 2005; **41:** 321–27.

88. Barengo NC, Sandstrom PH, Jormanainen VJ, Myllykangas MT. Changes in smoking prevalence among Finnish physicians 1990–2001. *Eur J Public Health* 2004; **14:** 201–03.

89. Kotz D, Wagena EJ, Wesseling G. Smoking cessation practices of Dutch general practitioners, cardiologists, and lung physicians. *Respir Med* 2007; **101:** 568–73.

90. Mohan S, Pradeepkumar AS, Thresia CU, Thankappan KR, Poston WS, Haddock CK, *et al.* Tobacco use among medical professionals in Kerala, India: the need for enhanced tobacco cessation and control efforts. *Addict Behav* 2006; **31:** 2313–18.

91. Ahmadi J, Khalili H, Jooybar R, Namazi N, Aghaei PM. Cigarette smoking among Iranian medical students, resident physicians and attending physicians. *Eur J Med Res* 2001; **6:** 406–08.

92. Power B, Neilson S, Perry IJ. Perception of the risks of smoking in the general population and among general practitioners in Ireland. *Ir J Med Sci* 2004; **173:** 141–44.

93. Franceschi S, Serraino D, Talamini R, Candiani E. Personal habits and attitudes towards smoking in a sample of physicians from the north-east of Italy. *Int J Epidemiol* 1986; **15:** 584–85.

94. Ficarra MG, Gualano MR, Capizzi S, Siliquini R, Liguori G, Manzoli L, *et al.* Tobacco use prevalence, knowledge and attitudes among Italian hospital healthcare professionals. *Eur J Public Health* 2010.

95. Kaneita Y, Uchida T, Ohida T. Epidemiological study of smoking among Japanese physicians. *Prev Med* 2010; **51:** 164–67.

96. Aaro LE, Bjartveit K, Vellar OD, Berglund EL. Smoking habits among Norwegian doctors 1974. *Scand J Soc Med* 1977; **5:** 127–35.

97. Saeed AA. Attitudes and behaviour of physicians towards smoking in Riyadh city, Saudi Arabia. *Trop Geogr Med* 1991; **43:** 76–79.

98. Sebo P, Bouvier Gallacchi M, Goehring C, Kunzi B, Bovier PA. Use of tobacco and alcohol by Swiss primary care physicians: a cross-sectional survey. *BMC Public Health* 2007; **7:** 5–8.

99. Sadowski IJ, Ruffieux C, Cornuz J. Self-reported smoking cessation activities among Swiss primary care physicians. *BMC Public Health* 2009; **10:** 1–6.

100. Akvardar Y, Demiral Y, Ergor G, Ergor A. Substance use among medical students and physicians in a medical school in Turkey. *Soc Psychiatry Psychiatr Epidemiol* 2004; **39:** 502–06.

101. Fowler G, Mant D, Fuller A, Jones L. The "Help Your Patient Stop" initiative. Evaluation of smoking prevalence and dissemination of WHO/UICC guidelines in UK general practice. *Lancet* 1989; **1:** 1253–55.

102. Hussain SF, Tjeder-Burton S, Campbell IA, Davies PD. Attitudes to smoking and smoking habits among hospital staff. *Thorax* 1993; **48:** 174–75.

103. Sachs DP. Smoking habits of pulmonary physicians. *N Engl J Med* 1983; **309:** 799.

104. Sachs DP. Treatment of cigarette dependency. What American pulmonary physicians do. *Am Rev Respir Dis* 1984; **129:** 1010–13.

105. Wells KB, Lewis CE, Leake B, Ware JE. Do physicians preach what they practice? A study of physicians' health habits and counseling practices. *JAMA* 1984; **252:** 2846–48.

106. Fortmann SP, Sallis JF, Magnus PM, Farquhar JW. Attitudes and practices of physicians regarding hypertension and smoking: The Stanford Five City Project. *Prev Med* 1985; **14:** 70–80.

107. Linn LS, Yager J, Cope D, Leake B. Health habits and coping behaviors among practicing physicians. *West J Med* 1986; **144:** 484–89.

108. Hughes PH, Brandenburg N, Baldwin DC, Storr CL, Williams KM, Anthony JC. Prevalence of substance use among US physicians. *JAMA* 1992; **267:** 2333–39.

109. Hensrud DD, Sprafka JM. The smoking habits of Minnesota physicians. *Am J Pub Health* 1993; **83:** 415–17.

110. Hepburn MJ, Johnson JM, Ward JA, Longfield JN. A survey of smoking cessation knowledge, training, and practice among U.S. Army general medical officers. *Am J Prev Med* 2000; **18:** 300–04.

111. Misra R, Vadaparampil ST. Personal cancer prevention and screening practices among Asian Indian physicians in the United States. *Cancer Detect Prev* 2004; **28:** 269–76.

112. Allard RH. Tobacco and oral health: attitudes and opinions of European dentists; a report of the EU working group on tobacco and oral health. *Int Dent J* 2000; **50:** 99–102.

113. Halling A, Uhrbom E, Bjerner B, Solen G. Tobacco habits, attitudes and participating behavior in tobacco prevention among dental personnel in Sweden. *Community Dent Oral Epidemiol* 1995; **23:** 254–55.

114. Christen AG. Survey of smoking behavior and attitudes of 630 American dentists: current trends. *J Am Dent Assoc* 1984; **109:** 271–72.

115. Rodrigues GA, Galvao V, Viegas CA. Prevalence of smoking among dentists in the Federal District of Brasilia, Brazil. *J Bras Pneumol* 2008; **34:** 288–93.

116. Laskin DM. Smoking habits and attitudes of oral and maxillofacial surgeons. *J Oral Maxillofac Surg* 1987; **45:** 493–95.

117. Mullins R. Attitudes and smoking habits of dentists in Victoria: 16 years on. *Aust Dent J* 1994; **39:** 324–26.

118. Lodi G, Bez C, Rimondini L, Zuppiroli A, Sardella A, Carrassi A. Attitude towards smoking and oral cancer prevention among northern Italian dentists. *Oral Oncol* 1997; **33:** 100–04.

119. Burgan SZ. Smoking behavior and views of Jordanian dentists: A pilot survey. *Oral Surg Oral Med Oral Pathol Oral Radiol Endod* 2003; **95:** 163–68.

120. Leggat PA, Chowanadisai S, Kedjarune U, Kukiattrakoon B, Yapong B. Health of dentists in southern Thailand. *Int Dent J* 2001; **51:** 348–52.

121. Clover K, Hazell T, Stanbridge V, Sanson-Fisher R. Dentists' attitudes and practice regarding smoking. *Aust Dent J* 1999; **44:** 46–50.

122. Ayers KM, Thomson WM, Newton JT, Morgaine KC, Rich AM. Self-reported occupational health of general dental practitioners. *Occup Med (Lond)* 2009; **59:** 142–48.

123. Campbell HS, Macdonald JM. Tobacco counselling among Alberta dentists. *J Can Dent Assoc* 1994; **60:** 218–20, 23–26.

124. Nishio N, Kouda K, Nishio J, Nakamura H, Sonoda Y, Takeshita T. Smoking prevalence among dentists in Hyogo, Japan 2003. *Ind Health* 2009; **47:** 431–35.

125. Ghasemi H, Murtomaa H, Vehkalahti MM, Torabzadeh H. Determinants of oral health behaviour among Iranian dentists. *Int Dent J* 2007; **57:** 237–42.

126. Skegg JA, McGee RO, Stewart AW. Smoking prevention: attitudes and activities of New Zealand dentists. *NZ Dent J* 1995; **91:** 4–7.

127. Gorter RC, Eijkman MA, Hoogstraten J. Burnout and health among Dutch dentists. *Eur J Oral Sci* 2000; **108:** 261–67.

128. McCartan BE, Sadlier D, O'Mullane DM. Smoking habits and attitudes of Irish dentists and dental students. *J Ir Dent Assoc* 1993; **39:** 26–29.

129. Piedro EC, Romero SO, Sala EC. Prevalence of smoking among dentists in Catalonia – Spain (2006). Literature review of smoking cessation practices in the dental office. *Med Oral Pathol Oral Cir Bucal* 2008; **13:** 671–77.

130. Smith DR, Leggat PA. Tobacco smoking prevalence among a cross-section of dentists in Queensland, Australia. *Kurume Med J* 2005; **52:** 147–51.

131. Fried JL, Cohen LA. Maryland dentists' attitudes regarding tobacco issues. *Clin Prev Dent* 1992; **14:** 10–16.

132. John JH, Thomas D, Richards D. Smoking cessation interventions in the Oxford region: changes in dentists' attitudes and reported practices 1996–2001. *Br Dent J* 2003; **195:** 270–75.

133. John JH, Yudkin P, Murphy M, Ziebland S, Fowler GH. Smoking cessation interventions for dental patients – attitudes and reported practices of dentists in the Oxford region. *Br Dent J* 1997; **183:** 359–64.

134. Secker–Walker RH, Solomon LJ, Hill HC. A statewide survey of dentists' smoking cessation advice. *J Am Dent Assoc* 1989; **118:** 37–40.

135. Lund M, Lund KE, Rise J. Preventing tobacco use in Norwegian dental practice. *Community Dent Oral Epidemiol* 2004; **32:** 385–94.

136. Kay EJ, Scarrott DM. A survey of dental professionals' health and well-being. *Br Dent J* 1997; **183:** 340–45.

137. O'Shea RM, Corah NL. The dentist's role in cessation of cigarette smoking. *Public Health Rep* 1984; **99:** 510–14.

138. Hastreiter RJ, Bakdash B, Roesch MH, Walseth J. Use of tobacco prevention and cessation strategies and techniques in the dental office. *J Am Dent Assoc* 1994; **125:** 1475–84.

139. Logan H, Levy S, Ferguson K, Pomrehn P, Muldoon J. Tobacco-related attitudes and counseling practices of Iowa dentists. *Clin Prev Dent* 1992; **14:** 19–22.

140. Underwood B, Fox K, Nixon PJ. Alcohol and drug use among vocational dental practitioners. *Br Dent J* 2003; **195:** 265–68; discussion 59.

141. Telivuo M, Vehkalahti M, Lahtinen A, Murtomaa H. Finnish dentists as tobacco counselors. *Community Dent Oral Epidemiol* 1991; **19:** 221–24.

142. Albert DA, Severson H, Gordon J, Ward A, Andrews J, Sadowsky D. Tobacco attitudes, practices, and behaviors: a survey of dentists participating in managed care. *Nicotine Tob Res* 2005; **7 Suppl 1:** S9–18.

143. Tomar SL. Dentistry's role in tobacco control. *J Am Dent Assoc* 2001; **132 Suppl:** 30S–35S.

144. Tomar SL, Husten CG, Manley MW. Do dentists and physicians advise tobacco users to quit? *J Am Dent Assoc* 1996; **127:** 259–65.

145. Kunzel C, Lalla E, Albert DA, Yin H, Lamster IB. On the primary care frontlines: the role of the general practitioner in smoking-cessation activities and diabetes management. *J Am Dent Assoc* 2005; **136:** 1144–53; quiz 67.

146. Glick M. Smoking cessation: no longer a choice. *J Am Dent Assoc* 2005; **136:** 1076, 1078.

147. Christen AG. Tobacco cessation, the dental profession, and the role of dental education. *J Dent Educ* 2001; **65**: 368–74.

148. Dodds AM, Gray NJ, Hill DJ, Rankin DW. Attitudes and smoking habits of dentists in Victoria. *Aust Dent J* 1979; **24**: 143–45.

149. Trotter L, Worcester P. Training for dentists in smoking cessation intervention. *Aust Dent J* 2003; **48**: 183–89.

150. Chestnutt IG, Binnie VI. Smoking cessation counselling – a role for the dental profession? *Br Dent J* 1995; **179**: 411–15.

151. Newbury-Birch D, Lowry RJ, Kamali F. The changing patterns of drinking, illicit drug use, stress, anxiety and depression in dental students in a UK dental school: a longitudinal study. *Br Dent J* 2002; **192**: 646–49.

152. Merchant A, Pitiphat W, Douglass CW, Crohin C, Joshipura K. Oral hygiene practices and periodontitis in health care professionals. *J Periodontol* 2002; **73**: 531–35.

153. Myers AH, Rosner B, Abbey H, Willet W, Stampfer MJ, Bain C, Lipnick R, Hennekens C, Speizer F. Smoking behavior among participants in the nurses' health study. *Am J Public Health* 1987; **77**: 628–30.

154. Bain C, Feskanich D, Speizer FE, Thun M, Hertzmark E, Rosner BA, Colditz GA. Lung cancer rates in men and women with comparable histories of smoking. *J Natl Cancer Inst* 2004; **96**: 826–34.

155. Harrison MB. Assessment of the smoking prevention and cessation needs of Canadian student nurses & registered nurses. *Can J Cardiovasc Nurs* 1991; **2**: 22.

156. John U, Hanke M. Tobacco-smoking prevalence among physicians and nurses in countries with different tobacco-control activities. *Eur J Cancer Prev* 2003; **12**: 235–37.

157. Steptoe A, Doherty S, Kendrick T, Rink E, Hilton S. Attitudes to cardiovascular health promotion among GPs and practice nurses. *Fam Pract* 1999; **16**: 158–63.

158. Smith DR, Wei N, Wang RS. Contemporary smoking habits among nurses in Mainland China. *Contemp Nurse* 2005; **20**: 258–66.

159. Yang MS, Yang MJ, Pan SM. Prevalence and correlates of substance use among clinical nurses in Kaohsiung city. *Kaohsiung J Med Sci* 2001; **17**: 261–69 [in Chinese].

160. Alexander LL, Beck K. The smoking behaviour of military nurses: the relationship to job stress, job satisfaction and social support. *J Adv Nurs* 1990; **15**: 843–49.

161. Petch-Levine D, Young Cureton V, Canham D, Murray M. Health practices of school nurses. *J Sch Nurs* 2003; **19**: 273–80.

162. Sekijima K, Seki N, Suzuki H. Smoking prevalence and attitudes toward tobacco among student and staff nurses in Niigata, Japan. *Tohoku J Exp Med* 2005; **206**: 187–94.

163. Alderman C. Here's looking at you. *Nurs Stand* 1997; **11**: 23–27.

164. Gray J. Number of nurses who smoke 'extremely low'. *Nurs Stand* 1997; **11:** 5.

165. Johnston JM, Chan SS, Chan SK, Lam TH, Chi I, Leung GM. Training nurses and social workers in smoking cessation counseling: a population needs assessment in Hong Kong. *Prev Med* 2005; **40:** 389–406.

166. Ernster V, Kaufman N, Nichter M, Samet J, Yoon SY. Women and tobacco: moving from policy to action. *Bull World Health Organ* 2000; **78:** 891–901.

167. Mackay J. Women and tobacco: international issues. *J Am Med Womens Assoc* 1996; **51:** 48–51.

168. Reeve K, Adams J, Kouzekanani K. The nurse as exemplar: smoking status as a predictor of attitude toward smoking and smoking cessation. *Cancer Pract* 1996; **4:** 31–33.

169. Sarna LP, Brown JK, Lillington L, Rose M, Wewers ME, Brecht ML. Tobacco interventions by oncology nurses in clinical practice: report from a national survey. *Cancer* 2000; **89:** 881–89.

170. Yankie VM, Price HM, Nanfito ER, Jasinski DM, Crowell NA, Heath J. Providing smoking cessation counseling: a national survey among nurse anesthetists. *Crit Care Nurs Clin North Am* 2006; **18:** 123–29, xiv.

171. Beletsioti-Stika P, Scriven A. Smoking among Greek nurses and their readiness to quit. *Int Nurs Rev* 2006; **53:** 150–56.

172. Kaplan B, Yogev Y, Fisher M, Gall B, Dekel A, Sulkes J, Rabinerson D. Self-health attitudes and practices of obstetrics and gynecology nurses in Israel. *Clin Exp Obstet Gynecol* 2002; **29:** 115–16.

173. Sezer H, Guler N, Sezer RE. Smoking among nurses in Turkey: comparison with other countries. *J Health Popul Nutr* 2007; **25:** 107–11.

174. Kirkby RJ, Bashkawi EB, Drew CA, Foenander GP. Smoking in nurses. *Med J Aust* 1976; **2:** 864–65.

175. Hughes AM, Rissel C. Smoking: rates and attitudes among nursing staff in central Sydney. *Int J Nurs Pract* 1999; **5:** 147–54.

176. Chalmers K, Bramadat IJ, Cantin B, Murnaghan D, Shuttleworth E, Scott-Findlay S, Tataryn D. A smoking reduction and cessation program with registered nurses: findings and implications for community health nursing. *J Community Health Nurs* 2001; **18:** 115–34.

177. Morra ME, Knobf MK. Comparison of nurses' smoking habits: the 1975 DHEW survey and Connecticut nurses, 1981. *Public Health Rep* 1983; **98:** 553–57.

178. Nelson DE, Giovino GA, Emont SL, Brackbill R, Cameron LL, Peddicord J. Trends in cigarette smoking among US physicians and nurses. *JAMA* 1994; **271:** 1273–75.

179. Ohida T, Osaki Y, Kobayashi Y, Sekiyama M, Minowa M. Smoking prevalence of female nurses in the national hospitals of Japan. *Tob Control* 1999; **8:** 192–95.

180. Kitajima T, Ohida T, Harano S, Kamal AM, Takemura S, Nozaki N, Kawahara K, Minaowa M.

Smoking behavior, initiating and cessation factors among Japanese nurses: a cohort study. *Public Health* 2002; **116:** 347–52.

181. Smith DR, Adachi Y, Mihashi M, Ueno C, Ishitake T. Tobacco smoking habits among a cross-section of rural Japanese nurses. *Aust J Adv Nurs* 2006; **24:** 33–37.

182. Spencer JK. Nurses' cigarette smoking in England and Wales. *Int J Nurs Stud* 1984; **21:** 69–79.

183. Blakey R, Seaton A. Smoking attitudes amongst nursing tutors and their students. *Health Bull (Edinb)* 1992; **50:** 417–21.

184. Dickens GL, Stubbs JH, Haw CM. Smoking and mental health nurses: a survey of clinical staff in a psychiatric hospital. *J Psychiatr Ment Health Nurs* 2004; **11:** 445–51.

185. Stubbs J, Haw C, Garner L. Survey of staff attitudes to smoking in a large psychiatric hospital. *Psychiatric Bull* 2004; **28:** 204–07.

186. Bloor RN, Meeson L, Crome IB. The effects of a non-smoking policy on nursing staff smoking behaviour and attitudes in a psychiatric hospital. *J Psychiatr Ment Health Nurs* 2006; **13:** 188–96.

187. Hay DR. The smoking habits of nurses in New Zealand: results from the 1976 population census. *NZ Med J* 1980; **92:** 391–93.

188. Ohida T, Kawahara K, Osaki Y, Sone T, Kamal AM, Kawaguchi T, Sekiyama M, Harita A, Minowa M. Behaviors and attitudes towards smoking among the nurses in Japan. *J Epidemiol* 2000; **10:** 344–48.

189. Group UNITEUS. A survey of coronary risk factors in a cohort of cardiac nurses from Europe: Do nurses practise what they preach? *Eur J Cardiovasc Nurs* 2002; **1:** 57–60.

190. Plant ML, Plant MA, Foster J. Alcohol, tobacco and illicit drug use amongst nurses: a Scottish study. *Drug Alcohol Depend* 1991; **28:** 195–202.

191. Fernandez D, Martin V, Molina AJ, De Luis JM. Smoking habits of students of nursing: a questionnaire survey (2004–2006). *Nurse Educ Today* 2010; **30:** 480–84.

192. Jones TE, Crocker H, Ruffin RE. Smoking habits and cessation programme in an Australian teaching hospital. *Aust NZ J Med* 1998; **28:** 446–52.

193. Nagle A, Schofield M, Redman S. Australian nurses' smoking behaviour, knowledge and attitude towards providing smoking cessation care to their patients. *Health Promot Int*1999; **14:** 133–44.

194. Dore K, Hoey J. Smoking practices, knowledge and attitudes regarding smoking of university hospital nurses. *Can J Public Health* 1988; **79:** 170–74.

195. O'Connor AM, Harrison M. Survey of smoking prevalence among Canadian nursing students and registered nurses. *Can J Public Health* 1992; **83:** 417–21.

196. Chalmers K, Bramadat IJ, Cantin B, Shuttleworth E, Scott-Findlay S. Smoking characteristics of Manitoba nurses. *Can Nurse* 2000; **96:** 31–34.

197. Pelkonen M, Kankkunen P. Nurses' competence in advising and supporting clients to cease smoking: a survey among Finnish nurses. *J Clin Nurs* 2001; **10:** 437–41.

198. Cooreman J, Pretet S, Levallois M, Marsac J, Perdrizet S. Smoking among hospital nurses. *Am J Public Health* 1989; **79:** 782.

199. Tselebis A, Panaghiotou A, Theotoka I, Ilias I. Nursing staff anxiety versus smoking habits. *Int J Nurs Pract* 2001; **7:** 221–23.

200. Callaghan P, Fun MK, Yee FC. Hong Kong nurses' health-related behaviours: implications for nurses' role in health promotion. *J Adv Nurs* 1997; **25:** 1276–82.

201. Ota A, Yasuda N, Okamoto Y, Kobayashi Y, Sugihara Y, Koda S, Kawakami N, Ohara H. Relationship of job stress with nicotine dependence of smokers – a cross-sectional study of female nurses in a general hospital. *J Occup Health* 2004; **46:** 220-24.

202. Retief FW, Prinsloo E, Calitz J, Barnes JM. Smoking among nursing staff at Tygerberg Hospital, Cape Town. *S Afr Med J* 2003; **93:** 661–63.

203. Hope A, Kelleher CC, O'Connor M. Lifestyle practices and the health promoting environment of hospital nurses. *J Adv Nurs* 1998; **28:** 438–47.

204. Rowe K, Clark JM. Evaluating the effectiveness of a smoking cessation intervention designed for nurses. *Int J Nurs Stud* 1999; **36:** 301–11.

205. McKenna H, Slater P, McCance T, Bunting B, Spiers A, McElwee G. The role of stress, peer influence and education levels on the smoking behaviour of nurses. *Int J Nurs Stud* 2003; **40:** 359–66.

206. Feldman R. Smoking and the psych nurse. *J Psychosoc Nurs Ment Health Serv* 1984; **22:** 13–16.

207. Becker DM, Myers AH, Sacci M, Weida S, Swank R, Levine DM, Pearson TA. Smoking behavior and attitudes toward smoking among hospital nurses. *Am J Public Health* 1986; **76:** 1449–51.

208. Brown MH, Kiss ME. Evaluation of competition as a method to recruit nurses into an employee self-help quit-smoking program. A failed experiment. *Cancer Nurs* 1987; **10:** 227–30.

209. Haughey BP, Kuhn MA, Dittmar SS, Wu YW. Health practices of critical care nurses. *Heart Lung* 1992; **21:** 203–08.

210. Stillman FA, Hantula DA, Swank R. Creating a smoke-free hospital: attitudes and smoking behaviors of nurses and physicians. *Am J Health Promot* 1994; **9:** 108–14.

211. Mundt MH, Glass LK, Michaels C. A professional challenge: nurses and smoking. *J Community Health Nurs* 1995; **12:** 139–46.

212. Blazer LK, Mansfield PK. A comparison of substance use rates among female nurses, clerical workers and blue-collar workers. *J Adv Nurs* 1995; **21:** 305–13.

213. Trinkoff AM, Storr CL. Substance use among nurses: differences between specialties. *Am J Public Health* 1998; **88:** 581–85.

214. Collins RL, Gollnisch G, Morsheimer ET. Substance use among a regional sample of female nurses. *Drug Alcohol Depend* 1999; **55:** 145–55.

215. Barrett TW, Norton VC, Busam M, Boyd J, Maron DJ, Slovis CM. Self-reported cardiac risk factors in emergency department nurses and paramedics. *Prehosp Disaster Med* 2000; **15:** 14–17.

216. Borrelli B, Hecht JP, Papandonatos GD, Emmons KM, Tatewosian LR, Abrams DB. Smoking-cessation counseling in the home. Attitudes, beliefs, and behaviors of home healthcare nurses. *Am J Prev Med* 2001; **21:** 272–77.

217. Braun BL, Fowles JB, Solberg LI, Kind EA, Lando H, Pine D. Smoking-related attitudes and clinical practices of medical personnel in Minnesota. *Am J Prev Med* 2004; **27:** 316–22.

218. Brown DE, James GD, Mills PS. Occupational differences in job strain and physiological stress: female nurses and school teachers in Hawaii. *Psychosom Med* 2006; **68:** 524–30.

## Chapter 4


1. Moreno San-Pedro E, Roales-Nieto JG, Blanco-Coronado JL. Tobacco use among Spanish physicians and medical students. *Tob Control* 2006; **15:** 272.

2. Sockrider MM, Maguire GP, Haponik E, Davis A, Boehlecke B. Attitudes of respiratory care practitioners and students regarding pulmonary prevention. *Chest* 1998; **114:** 1193–98.

3. Baldwin DC, Jr., Hughes PH, Conard SE, Storr CL, Sheehan DV. Substance use among senior medical students. A survey of 23 medical schools. *JAMA* 1991; **265:** 2074–78.

4. Huy NV, An DTM, Phong DN. Smoking among Vietnamese medical students: Prevalence, costs, and predictors. *Asia Pac J Public Health* 2008; **20:** 16–24.

5. Kocabas A, Burgut R, Bozdemir Nk, A, , Cildag O, Dagli E, Erkan L, Isik R, Turktas H. Smoking patterns at different medical schools in Turkey. *Tob Control* 1994; **3:** 228–35.

6. Rodriguez ME, Cami J. Substance use among medical students in Barcelona (Spain). A comparison with previous surveys. *Drug Alcohol Depend* 1986; **18:** 311–18.

7. Rosselli D, Rey O, Calderon C, Rodriguez MN. Smoking in Colombian medical schools: the hidden curriculum. *Prev Med* 2001; **33:** 170–74.

8. Ahmadi J, Khalili H, Jooybar R, Namazi N, Aghaei PM. Cigarette smoking among Iranian medical students, resident physicians and attending physicians. *Eur J Med Res* 2001; **6:** 406–08.

9. Jarallah JS. Smoking habits of medical students at King Saud University, Riyadh. *Saudi Med J* 1992; **13:** 510–13.

10. Kawane H. Tobacco smoking in Japan. *Med J Aust* 1987; **146:** 503–04.

11. Kawane H. Antismoking education for medical students. *Chest* 1992; **101:** 1480.

12. Kusunoki T, Hosoi S, Asai K, Harazaki M, Furusho K. Relationships between atopy and lung function: results from a sample of one hundred medical students in Japan. *Ann Allergy Asthma Immunol* 1999; **83:** 343–47.

13. Merrill JR, Madanat HN, Cox E, Merrill JM. Perceived effectiveness of counselling patients about smoking among medical students in Amman, Jordan. *East Mediterr Health J* 2009; **15:** 1180–91.

14. Roy M, Chakraborty AK. Smoking and drug-abuse among the newly admitted students of medical colleges in West Bengal. *Indian J Public Health* 1981; **25:** 30–35.

15. Webb E, Ashton CH, Kelly P, Kamah F. An update on British medical students' lifestyles. *Med Educ* 1998; **32:** 325–31.

16. Wong ML, Chen PC. Smoking behaviour, knowledge and opinion of medical students. *Med J Malaysia* 1989; **44:** 317–23.

17. Yaacob I, Abdullah ZA. Smoking behavior, knowledge and opinion of medical students. *Asia Pac J Public Health* 1994; **7:** 88–91.

18. Conard S, Hughes P, Baldwin DC, Jr., Achenbach KE, Sheehan DV. Substance use by fourth-year students at 13 U.S. medical schools. *J Med Educ* 1988; **63:** 747–58.

19. Lam TS, Tse LA, Yu IT, Griffiths S. Prevalence of smoking and environmental tobacco smoke exposure, and attitudes and beliefs towards tobacco control among Hong Kong medical students. *Public Health* 2009; **123:** 42–46.

20. Patkar AA, Hill K, Batra V, Vergare MJ, Leone FT. A comparison of smoking habits among medical and nursing students. *Chest* 2003; **124:** 1415–20.

21. Mangus RS, Hawkins CE, Miller MJ. Tobacco and alcohol use among 1996 medical school graduates. *JAMA* 1998; **280:** 1192–93, 95.

22. Richmond RL, Kehoe L. Smoking behaviour and attitudes among Australian medical students. *Med Educ* 1997; **31:** 169–76.

23. Daudt AW, Alberg AJ, Prola JC, Fialho L, Petracco A, Wilhelms A, Weiss A, Estery C. A first step incorporating smoking education into a Brazilian medical school curriculum: results of a survey to assess the cigarette smoking knowledge, attitudes, behaviour, and clinical practices of medical students. *J Addict Dis* 1999; **18:** 19–29.

24. Lei Z, Jingheng H, Jianzhong L. Smoking among Shanghai medical students and the need for comprehensive intervention strategies. *Health Promot Int* 1997; **12:** 27–32.

25. Centers for Disease Control and Prevention (CDC). Tobacco use and cessation counseling – global health professionals survey pilot study, 10 countries, 2005. *MMWR Morb Mortal Wkly Rep* 2005; **54:** 505–09.

26. Franca LR, Dautzenberg B, Falissard B, Reynaud M. Peer substance use overestimation among French university students: a cross-sectional survey. *BMC Public Health* 2010; **10:** 169.

27. Ramakrishna GS, Sankara Sarma P, Thankappan KR. Tobacco use among medical students in Orissa. *Natl Med J India* 2005; **18:** 285–89.

28. Engs RC. The drug-use patterns of helping-profession students in Brisbane, Australia. *Drug Alcohol Depend* 1980; **6:** 231–46.

29. Roche AM. Have efforts to improve medical students' drug and alcohol knowledge, skills and attitudes worked? *Drug Alcohol Rev* 1997; **16:** 157–70.

30. Roche AM, Beauchamp P. Smoking prevalence among senior medical students. *Med J Aust* 1994; **160:** 447–48.

31. Roche AM, Eccleston P, Jordan D. Smoking-related knowledge and attitudes of senior Australian medical students. *Tob Control* 1996; **5:** 271–79.

32. Thakore S, Ismail Z, Jarvis S, Payne E, Keetbaas S, Payne R, Rothenburg L. The perceptions and habits of alcohol consumption and smoking among Canadian medical students. *Acad Psychiatry* 2009; **33:** 193–97.

33. Smith DR, Wei N, Wang RS. Tobacco smoking habits among Chinese medical students and their need for health promotion initiatives. *Health Promot J Austr* 2005; **16:** 233–35.

34. Behera D, Malik SK. Smoking habit of undergraduate medical students. *Indian J Chest Dis Allied Sci* 1987; **29:** 182–84.

35. Songkla YN, Saenghirunvattana S. Smoking among medical students. *J Med Assoc Thai* 1985; **68:** 198–200.

36. Najem GR, Passannante MR, Foster JD. Health risk factors and health promoting behavior of medical, dental and nursing students. *J Clin Epidemiol* 1995; **48:** 841–49.

37. Frisch AS, Kurtz M, Shamsuddin K. Knowledge, attitudes and preventive efforts of Malaysian medical students regarding exposure to environmental tobacco and cigarette smoking. *J Adolesc* 1999; **22:** 627–34.

38. Minhas HM, Rahman A. Prevalence, patterns and knowledge of effects on health of smoking among medical students in Pakistan. *East Mediterr Health J* 2009; **15:** 1174–79.

39. Sichletidis LT, Chloros D, Tsiotsios I, Kottakis I, Kaiafa O, Kaouri S, Karamanlidis A, Kalkanis D, Posporelis S. High prevalence of smoking in Northern Greece. *Prim Care Respir J* 2006; **15:** 92–97.

40. Sezer H, Guler N, Sezer RE. Smoking among nurses in Turkey: comparison with other countries. *J Health Popul Nutr* 2007; **25:** 107–11.

41. Piko BF. Does knowledge count? Attitudes toward smoking among medical, nursing, and pharmacy students in Hungary. *J Community Health* 2002; **27:** 269–76.

42. Kavcova E, Kocan I, Squier C. Tobacco control and the role of the medical community in the Slovak Republic. *Eur J Dent Educ* 2004; **8 Suppl 4:** 46–50.

43. Melani AS, Verponziani W, Boccoli E, Trianni GL, Federici A, Amerini R, Vichi MG, Sestini P. Tobacco smoking habits, attitudes and beliefs among nurse and medical students in Tuscany. *Eur J Epidemiol* 2000; **16:** 607–11.

44. Xiang H, Wang Z, Stallones L, Yu S, Gimbel HW, Yang P. Cigarette smoking among medical college students in Wuhan, People's Republic of China. *Prev Med* 1999; **29:** 210–15.

45. Al-Haqwi AL, Tamim H, Asery A. Knowledge, attitude and practice of tobacco smoking by medical students in Riyadh, Saudi Arabia. *Ann Thorac Med* 2010; **5:** 145–48.

46. Ernster V, Kaufman N, Nichter M, Samet J, Yoon SY. Women and tobacco: moving from policy to action. *Bull World Health Organ* 2000; **78:** 891–901.

47. Richmond R. Teaching medical students about tobacco. *Thorax* 1999; **54:** 70–78.

48. Ahmed EN, Jafarey NA. Smoking habits amongst medical students of Sind Medical College. *J Pak Med Assoc* 1983; **33:** 39–44.

49. Mubeen SM, Morrow M, Barraclough S. Smoking among future doctors in a "no-smoking" university campus in Karachi, Pakistan: issues of tobacco control. *J Pak Med Assoc* 2008; **58:** 248–53.

50. Harrabi I, Ghannem H, Kacem M, Gaha R, Ben Abdelaziz A, Tessier JF. Medical students and tobacco in 2004: a survey in Sousse, Tunisia. *Int J Tuberc Lung Dis* 2006; **10:** 328–32.

51. Singh SK, Narang RK, Chandra S, Chaturvedi PK, Dubey AL. Smoking habits of the medical students. *Indian J Chest Dis Allied Sci* 1989; **31:** 99–103.

52. Elkind AK. Changes in the smoking behaviour, knowledge and opinion of medical students, 1972–1981. *Soc Sci Med* 1982; **16:** 2137–43.

53. Vlajinac H, Adanja B, Jarebinski M. Cigarette smoking among medical students in Belgrade related to parental smoking habits. *Soc Sci Med* 1989; **29:** 891–94.

54. Venkataraman S, Mukhopadhya A, Muliyil J. Trends of smoking among medical students. *Indian J Med Res* 1996; **104:** 316–20.

55. Boland M, Fitzpatrick P, Scallan E, Daly L, Herity B, Horgan J, Bourke G. Trends in medical student use of tobacco, alcohol and drugs in an Irish university, 1973–2002. *Drug Alcohol Depend* 2006; **85:** 123–28.

56. Ozasa K, Shigeta M, Hayashi K, Yuge M, Watanabe Y. Smoking prevalence in Japanese medical students, 1992–2004. *Med Educ* 2005; **39:** 971–72.

57. Senol Y, Donmez L, Turkay M, Aktekin M. The incidence of smoking and risk factors for smoking initiation in medical faculty students: cohort study. *BMC Public Health* 2006; **6:** 128.

58. Vakeflliu Y, Argjiri D, Peposhi I, Agron S, Melani AS. Tobacco smoking habits, beliefs, and attitudes among medical students in Tirana, Albania. *Prev Med* 2002; **34:** 370–73.

59. Roche AM, Eccleston P, Sanson-Fisher R. Teaching smoking cessation skills to senior medical students: a block-randomized controlled trial of four different approaches. *Prev Med* 1996; **25:** 251–58.

60. Roche AM, Sanson-Fisher RW, Cockburn J. Training experiences immediately after medical school. *Med Educ* 1997; **31:** 9–16.

61. Paine PA, Amaral JA, Pereira MG. Association between parental and student smoking behaviour in a Brazilian medical school. *Int J Epidemiol* 1985; **14:** 330–32.

62. Stramari LM, Kurtz M, Silva LC. Prevalence of and variables related to smoking among medical students at a university in the city of Passo Fundo, Brazil. *J Bras Pneumol* 2009; **35:** 442–48.

63. Trkulja V, Zivcec Z, Cuk M, Lackovic Z. Use of psychoactive substances among Zagreb University medical students: follow-up study. *Croat Med J* 2003; **44:** 50–58.

64. Brenner H, Scharrer S. Smoking habits of future physicians: a survey among medical students of a south German university. *Soz Praventivmed* 1996; **41:** 150–57.

65. Kusma B, Quarcoo D, Vitzthum K, Welte T, Mache S, Meyer-Falcke A, Groneberg DA, Raupach T. Berlin's medical students' smoking habits, knowledge about smoking and attitudes toward smoking cessation counseling. *J Occup Med Toxicol* 2010; **5:** 9.

66. Mammas IN, Bertsias GK, Linardakis M, Tzanakis NE, Labadarios DN, Kafatos AG. Cigarette smoking, alcohol consumption, and serum lipid profile among medical students in Greece. *Eur J Public Health* 2003; **13:** 278–82.

67. Alexopoulos EC, Jelastopulu E, Aronis K, Dougenis D. Cigarette smoking among university students in Greece: a comparison between medical and other students. *Environ Health Prev Med* 2010; **15:** 115–20.

68. Waalkens HJ, Cohen Schotanus J, Adriaanse H, Knol K. Smoking habits in medical students and physicians in Groningen, The Netherlands. *Eur Respir J* 1992; **5:** 49–52.

69. Dekker HM, Looman CWN, Adriaanse HP, Van Der Maas PJ. Prevalence of smoking in physicians and medical students, and the generation effect in the Netherlands. *Soc Sci Med* 1993; **36:** 817–22.

70. Piko B, Barabas K, Markos J. Health risk behaviour of a medical student population: report on a pilot study. *J R Soc Health* 1996; **116:** 97–100.

71. Singh G, Singh R, Jindal KC. Drug use among physicians and medical students. *Indian J Med Res* 1981; **73:** 594–602.

72. Sandell J, Singh S, Sati TK, Mehrotra SK. A study of smoking habits of medical students of Uttar Pradesh. *Indian J Public Health* 1983; **27:** 96–101.

73. Sinha DN, Gupta PC. Tobacco and areca nut use in male medical students of Patna. *Natl Med J India* 2001; **14:** 176–78.

74. Mohan S, Pradeepkumar AS, Thresia CU, Thankappan KR, Poston WS, Haddock CK, *et al.* Tobacco use among medical professionals in Kerala, India: the need for enhanced tobacco cessation and control efforts. *Addict Behav* 2006; **31:** 2313–18.

75. Sinha DN, Singh G, Gupta PC, Pednekar M, Warrn CW, Asma S, Lee J. Linking India global health professions student survey data to the World Health Organization framework convention on tobacco control. *Indian J Cancer* 2010; **47 Suppl 1:** 30–34.

76. Ficarra MG, Gualano MR, Capizzi S, Siliquini R, Liguori G, Manzoli L, *et al.* Tobacco use prevalence, knowledge and attitudes among Italian hospital healthcare professionals. *Eur J Public Health* 2010.

77. Tamaki T, Kaneita Y, Ohida T, Yokoyama E, Osaki Y, Kanda H, Takemura S, Hayashi K. Prevalence of and factors associated with smoking among Japanese medical students. *J Epidemiol* 2010; **20:** 339–45.

78. Komu P, Dimba EA, Macigo FG, Ogwell AE. Cigarette smoking and oral health among healthcare students. *East Afr Med J* 2009; **86:** 178–82.

79. Hussain SF, Moid I, Khan JA. Attitudes of Asian medical students towards smoking. *Thorax* 1995; **50:** 996–97.

80. Omair A, Kazmi T, Alam SE. Smoking prevalence and awareness about tobacco related diseases among medical students of Ziauddin Medical University. *J Pak Med Assoc* 2002; **52:** 389–92.

81. Khan FM, Husain SJ, Laeeq A, Awais A, Hussain SF, Khan JA. Smoking prevalence, knowledge and attitudes among medical students in Karachi, Pakistan. *East Mediterr Health J* 2005; **11:** 952–58.

82. Khan N, Siddiqui MU, Padhiar AA, Hashmi SAH, Fatima S, Muzaffar S. Prevalence, knowledge, attitude and practice of Shisha smoking among medical and dental students of Karachi, Pakistan. *J Dow Uni Health Sci* 2008; **2:** 3–10.

83. Al-Turki YA. Smoking habits among medical students in Central Saudi Arabia. *Saudi Med J* 2006; **27:** 700–03.

84. Almerie MQ, Matar HE, Salam M, Morad A, Abdulaal M, Koudsi A, Maziak W. Cigarettes and waterpipe smoking among medical students in Syria: a cross-sectional study. *Int J Tuberc Lung Dis* 2008; **12:** 1085–91.

85. Akvardar Y, Demiral Y, Ergor G, Ergor A, Bilici M, Akil Ozer O. Substance use in a sample of Turkish medical students. *Drug Alcohol Depend* 2003; **72:** 117–21.

86. Gulec M, Bakir B, Ozer M, Ucar M, Kilic S, Hasde M. Association between cigarette smoking and depressive symptoms among military medical students in Turkey. *Psychiatry Res* 2005; **134:** 281–86.

87. Birkner FE, Kunze M. Smoking patterns at a British and at an American medical school. *Med Educ* 1978; **12:** 128–32.

88. Ashton CH, Kamali F. Personality, lifestyles, alcohol and drug consumption in a sample of British medical students. *Med Educ* 1995; **29:** 187–92.

89. Engs RC, Van Teijlingen E. Correlates of alcohol, tobacco and marijuana use among Scottish postsecondary helping-profession students. *J Stud Alcohol* 1997; **58:** 435–44.

90. Ionescu C, Mihaescu T. Smoking behaviour, knowledge and attitudes of medicine, dentistry, and pharmacy students. *Rev Med Chir Soc Med Nat Iasi* 1986; **90:** 79–85.

91. Plasschaert AJ, Hoogstraten J, van Emmerik BJ, Webster DB, Clayton RR. Substance use among Dutch dental students. *Community Dent Oral Epidemiol* 2001; **29:** 48–54.

92. Khami MR, Murtomaa H, Razeghi S, Virtanen JI. Smoking and its determinants among Iranian dental students. *Med Princ Pract* 2010; **19:** 390–94.

93. de Andrade AP, Bernardo AC, Viegas CA, Ferreira DB, Gomes TC, Sales MR. Prevalence and characteristics of smoking among youth attending the University of Brasilia in Brazil. *J Bras Pneumol* 2006; **32:** 23–28.

94. Nagy K, Barabas K, Nyari T. Attitudes of Hungarian healthcare professional students to tobacco and alcohol. *Eur J Dent Educ* 2004; **8 Suppl 4:** 32–35.

95. Smith DR, Leggat PA, Walsh LJ. Workplace hazards among Australian dental students. *Aust Dent J* 2009; **54:** 186–88.

96. Tarlo SM, Sussman GL, Holness DL. Latex sensitivity in dental students and staff: a cross–sectional study. *J Allergy Clin Immunol* 1997; **99:** 396–401.

97. Victoroff KZ, Dankulich-Huryn T, Haque S. Attitudes of incoming dental students toward tobacco cessation promotion in the dental setting. *J Dent Educ* 2004; **68:** 563–68.

98. Barber MW, Fairclough A. A comparison of alcohol and drug use among dental undergraduates and a group of non-medical, professional undergraduates. *Br Dent J* 2006; **201:** 581–84; discussion 76.

99. Polychonopoulou A, Gatou T, Athanassouli T. Greek dental students' attitudes toward tobacco control programmes. *Int Dent J* 2004; **54:** 119–25.

100. Dumitrescu AL. Attitudes of Romanian dental students towards tobacco and alcohol. *J Contemp Dent Pract* 2007; **8:** 64–71.

101. Hennequin M, Tubert S, Devillers A, Muller M, Michailesco P, Peli JF, Pouezat J. Socio-economic and schooling status of dental undergraduates from six French universities. *Eur J Dent Educ* 2002; **6:** 95–103.

102. Olson DL, Shapiro S. Evaluation of smoking habits of dental students. *J Baltimore Coll Dent Surg* 1971; **26:** 40–44.

103. Olson DL, Shapiro S, Chellemi JS. Smoking habits of dental students. *J Baltimore Coll Dent Surg* 1970; **25:** 35–38.

104. Johansen JR. A survey of the periodontal conditions of dental students in India and Norway. *Acta Odontol Scand* 1970; **28:** 93–116.

105. Curson I, Manson JD. A study of a group of dental students, including their diet and dental health. *Br Dent J* 1965; **119:** 197–205.

106. Ashley MJ. Smoking habits, knowledge, and attitudes of final year university students in the health professions. *Prev Med* 1981; **10:** 645–54.

107. Sugiura G, Shinada K, Kawaguchi Y. Psychological well-being and perceptions of stress amongst Japanese dental students. *Eur J Dent Educ* 2005; **9:** 17–25.

108. Al-Omari Q, Barrieshi-Nusair K, Said K. Smoking prevalence and its effect on dental health attitudes and behavior among dental students. *Med Princ Pract* 2006; **15:** 195–99.

109. Al-Omari QD, Hamasha AA. Gender-specific oral health attitudes and behavior among dental students in Jordan. *J Contemp Dent Pract* 2005; **6:** 107–14.

110. Almas K, Al-Hawish A, Al-Khamis W. Oral hygiene practices, smoking habit, and self-perceived oral malodor among dental students. *J Contemp Dent Pract* 2003; **4:** 77–90.

111. Maatouk F, Maatouk W, Ghedira H, Ben Mimoun S. Effect of 5 years of dental studies on the oral health of Tunisian dental students. *East Mediterr Health J* 2006; **12:** 625–31.

112. Underwood B, Fox K. A survey of alcohol and drug use among UK based dental undergraduates. *Br Dent J* 2000; **189:** 314–17.

113. Newbury-Birch D, Lowry RJ, Kamali F. The changing patterns of drinking, illicit drug use, stress, anxiety and depression in dental students in a UK dental school: a longitudinal study. *Br Dent J* 2002; **192:** 646–49.

114. Kawamura M, Yip HK, Hu DY, Komabayashi T. A cross-cultural comparison of dental health attitudes and behaviour among freshman dental students in Japan, Hong Kong and West China. *Int Dent J* 2001; **51:** 159–63.

115. Smith DR, Leggat PA. A comparison of tobacco smoking among dentists in 15 countries. *Int Dent J* 2006; **56:** 283–88.

116. Smith DR, Leggat PA. An international review of tobacco smoking among medical students. *J Postgrad Med* 2007; **53:** 55–62.

117. Davis RM. When doctors smoke. *Tob Control* 1993; **2:** 187–88.

118. Rikard-Bell G, Groenlund C, Ward J. Australian dental students' views about smoking cessation counseling and their skills as counselors. *J Public Health Dent* 2003; **63:** 200–06.

119. Hussey DL, Burnett AC, Linden GJ. Characteristics of dental students in Ontario and Northern Ireland. *J Ir Dent Assoc* 1990; **36:** 133–35.

120. McCartan BE, Sadlier D, O'Mullane DM. Smoking habits and attitudes of Irish dentists and dental students. *J Ir Dent Assoc* 1993; **39:** 26–29.

121. Vered Y, Livny A, Zini A, Shabaita S, Sgan-Cohen HD. Dental students' attitudes and behavior toward smoking cessation as part of their professional education. *Teach Learn Med*; **22:** 268–73.

122. Gordon NA, Rayner CA. Smoking practices of dental and oral health students at the University of the Western Cape. *SADJ* 2010; **65:** 304–08.

123. Underwood B, Fox K, Manogue M. Tobacco, alcohol and drug use among dental undergraduates at one English university in 1998 and 2008. *Br Dent J* 2010; **208:** E8; discussion 164–65.

124. Yip JK, Hay JL, Ostroff JS, Stewart RK, Cruz GD. Dental students' attitudes toward smoking cessation guidelines. *J Dent Educ* 2000; **64:** 641–50.

125. Ahmadi J, Maharlooy N, Alishahi M. Substance abuse: prevalence in a sample of nursing students. *J Clin Nurs* 2004; **13:** 60–64.

126. Baron-Epel O, Josephsohn K, Ehrenfeld M. Nursing students' perceptions of smoking prevention. *Nurse Educ Today* 2004; **24:** 145–51.

127. Krommydas G, Kotrotsiou E, Raftopoulos V, Paralikas T, Gourgoulianis KI, Molyvdas PA. Smoking in health science students with asthma. *Can Respir J* 2004; **11**: 476.

128. Sekijima K, Seki N, Suzuki H. Smoking prevalence and attitudes toward tobacco among student and staff nurses in Niigata, Japan. *Tohoku J Exp Med* 2005; **206**: 187–94.

129. Suzuki K, Ohida T, Yokoyama E, Kaneita Y, Takemura S. Smoking among Japanese nursing students: nationwide survey. *J Adv Nurs* 2005; **49**: 268–75.

130. Blakey R, Seaton A. Smoking attitudes amongst nursing tutors and their students. *Health Bull (Edinb)* 1992; **50**: 417–21.

131. Boccoli E, Federici A, Melani AS, De Paola E. Results of a questionnaire about nurse students' smoking habits and knowledges in an Italian teaching school of nursing. *Eur J Epidemiol* 1996; **12**: 1–3.

132. Melani AS, Verponziani W, Boccoli E, Federici A, Sestini P. A comparison of smoking habits, beliefs and attitudes among Tuscan student nurses in 1992 and 1999. *Eur J Epidemiol* 2001; **17**: 417–21.

133. Carmichael A, Cockcroft A. Survey of student nurses' smoking habits in a London teaching hospital. *Respir Med* 1990; **84**: 277–82.

134. Clark E, McCann TV, Rowe K, Lazenbatt A. Cognitive dissonance and undergraduate nursing students' knowledge of, and attitudes about, smoking. *J Adv Nurs* 2004; **46**: 586–94.

135. O'Connor AM, Harrison M. Survey of smoking prevalence among Canadian nursing students and registered nurses. *Can J Public Health* 1992; **83**: 417–21.

136. Jenkins K, Ahijevych K. Nursing students' beliefs about smoking, their own smoking behaviors, and use of professional tobacco treatment intervention. *Appl Nurs Res* 2003; **16**: 164–72.

137. Sone T. Frequency of contact with cigarette advertising and smoking experience among young women in Japan. *J Epidemiol* 1997; **7**: 43–47.

138. Chalmers K, Seguire M, Brown J. Health promotion and tobacco control: student nurses' perspectives. *J Nurs Educ* 2003; **42**: 106–12.

139. Adams A, Bell PF, Pelletier SD. Nurses and smoking: a comparative study of students of nursing and teaching. *Aust Health Rev* 1994; **17**: 84–101.

140. Gorin SS. Predictors of tobacco control among nursing students. *Patient Educ Couns* 2001; **44**: 251–62.

141. Ohida T, Kamal AA, Takemura S, Sone T, Minowa M, Nozaki S. Smoking behavior and related factors among Japanese nursing students: a cohort study. *Prev Med* 2001; **32**: 341–47.

142. Shriver CB, Scott-Stiles A. Health habits of nursing versus non-nursing students: a longitudinal study. *J Nurs Educ* 2000; **39**: 308–14.

143. Boccoli E, Federici A, Trianni GL, Melani AS. Changes of smoking habits and beliefs during nurse training: a longitudinal study. *Eur J Epidemiol* 1997; **13**: 899–902.

144. Clement M, Jankowski LW, Bouchard L, Perreault M, Lepage Y. Health behaviors of nursing students: a longitudinal study. *J Nurs Educ* 2002; **41:** 257–65.

145. Sejr HS, Osler M. Do smoking and health education influence student nurses' knowledge, attitudes, and professional behavior? *Prev Med* 2002; **34:** 260–65.

146. Rowe K, Clark JM. Evaluating the effectiveness of a smoking cessation intervention designed for nurses. *Int J Nurs Stud* 1999; **36:** 301–11.

147. Hope A, Kelleher CC, O'Connor M. Lifestyle practices and the health promoting environment of hospital nurses. *J Adv Nurs* 1998; **28:** 438–47.

148. Neil JV, Clark D, Muller M. The smoking patterns and attitudes of student nurses and student teachers. *Aust Nurses J* 1980; **9:** 47–48.

149. Smith DR, Leggat PA. Tobacco smoking habits among a complete cross-section of Australian nursing students. *Nurs Health Sci* 2007; **9:** 82–89.

150. Zanetti F, Bergamaschi A, De Luca G, Stampi S. Tobacco smoking among nursing students: behaviour and knowledge of the correlated risks. *Ann Ig.* 2003; **15:** 545–50.

151. Biraghi E, Tortorano AM. Tobacco smoking habits among nursing students and the influence of family and peer smoking behaviour. *J Adv Nurs* 2010; **66:** 33–39.

152. Ohida T, Sakurai A, Kamal A, Sone T, Takemura S, Fukushima F. Smoking among Japanese nursing students: a nationwide survey. *Tob Control* 2001; **10:** 397.

153. Durmaz A, Üstün B. Determination of Smoking Habits and Personality Traits Among Nursing Students. *J Nurs Educ* 2006; **48:** 328–33.

154. Booth K, Faulkner A. Links between nurses and cigarette smoking? *Nurse Educ Today* 1986; **6:** 176–82.

155. West R, Hargreaves M. Factors associated with smoking in student nurses. *Psychol Health* 1995; **10:** 195–204.

156. Charlton A, While D, Mochizuki Y. A survey into the smoking habits of nursing students. *Nurs Times* 1997; **93:** 58–60.

157. Haughey BP, O'Shea RM, Dittmar SS, Bahn P, Mathewson M, Smith S, Brasure J. Smoking behavior among student nurses: a survey. *Public Health Rep.* 1986; **101:** 652–57.

## Chapter 5


1. 4,776 answer MM smoking survey. *Mod Med Aust.* August 1964 pp. 1–4.

2. Young JM, Ward JE. Implementing guidelines for smoking cessation advice in Australian general practice: opinions, current practices, readiness to change and perceived barriers. *Fam Pract* 2001; **18:** 14–20.

3. Nyman K. The health of general practitioners. A pilot survey. *Aust Fam Physician* 1991; **20:** 637–41, 44–45.

4. Roche AM, Parle MD, Stubbs JM, Hall W, Saunders JB. Management and treatment efficacy of drug and alcohol problems: What do doctors believe? *Addiction* 1995; **90:** 1357–66.

5. Dodds AM, Rankin DW, Hill DJ, Gray NJ. Attitudes and smoking habits of doctors in Victoria. *Community Health Stud* 1979; **3:** 28–31.

6. McCall L, Maher T, Piterman L. Preventive health behaviour among general practitioners in Victoria. *Aust Fam Physician* 1999; **28:** 854–57.

7. Rankin DW, Gray NJ, Hill DJ, Evans DR. Attitudes and smoking habits of Australian doctors. *Med J Aust* 1975; **2:** 822–24.

8. Roche AM, Parle MD, Saunders JB. Managing alcohol and drug problems in general practice: A survey of trainees' knowledge, attitudes and educational requirements. *Aust NZ J Public Health* 1996; **20:** 401–08.

9. Young JM, Ward JE. Declining rates of smoking among medical practitioners. *Med J Aust* 1997; **167:** 232.

10. You're setting the pace in the fitness stakes. *Med Pract.* September 1983 pp.22–24.

11. 5,976 answer MM smoking survey. *Mod Med Aust.* August 1970 pp.1–4.

12. Hill D, Borland R. Are doctors doing enough to stop their patients smoking? *Med J Aust* 1989; **150:** 413–14.

13. Dickinson JA, Wiggers J, Leeder SR, Sanson-Fisher RW. General practitioners' detection of patients' smoking status. *Med J Aust* 1989; **150:** 420–22, 5–6.

14. Chapman S, Wong WL, Smith W. Self-exempting beliefs about smoking and health: differences between smokers and ex-smokers. *Am J Public Health* 1993; **83:** 215–19.

15. Jones TE, Crocker H, Ruffin RE. Smoking habits and cessation programme in an Australian teaching hospital. *Aust NZ J Med* 1998; **28:** 446–52.

16. Glanz K, Fiel SB, Walker LR, Levy MR. Preventive health behavior of physicians. *J Med Educ* 1982; **57:** 637–39.

17. Samp RJ. Wisconsin physicians and cigarette smoking. *Wis Med J* 1963; **62:** 229.

18. Vaillant GE, Brighton JR, McArthur C. Physicians' use of mood-altering drugs. A 20-year follow-up report. *N Engl J Med* 1970; **282:** 365–70.

19. 60,000 answer MM smoking survey: Half of physicians don't smoke; nearly quarter use cigarettes. *Mod Med* 1964; **32:** 6, 18, 22, 30.

20. Scott HD, Tierney JT, Buechner JS, Waters WJ, Jr. Smoking rates among Rhode Island physicians: achieving a smoke-free society. *Am J Prev Med* 1992; **8:** 86–90.

21. Snegireff LS, Lombard OM. Comparative study of smoking habits of physicians. *N Engl J Med* 1955; **252:** 691–96.

22. Tate CI, Fulghum JE. Seventy per cent of Florida physicians are nonsmokers. *J Fla Med Assoc* 1965; **52:** 47–48.

23. Coe RM, Brehm HP. Smoking habits of physicians and preventive care practices. *HSMHA Health Rep* 1971; **86:** 217–21.

24. Eisinger RA. Cigarette smoking and the pediatrician. Findings based on a national survey. *Clin Pediatr (Phila)* 1972; **11:** 645–47.

25. Tamerin JS, Eisinger RA. Cigarette smoking and the psychiatrist. *Am J Psychiatry* 1972; **128:** 1224–29.

26. Fulghum JE, Groover ME, Jr., Williams AC, Braatz W. Smoking habits of Florida physicians revisited. *JFMA* 1972; **59:** 23–28.

27. Sachs DP. Smoking habits of pulmonary physicians. *N Engl J Med* 1983; **309:** 799.

28. Sachs DP. Treatment of cigarette dependency. What American pulmonary physicians do. *Am Rev Respir Dis* 1984; **129:** 1010–13.

29. Challberg K. Smoking habits of Rhode Island physicians. *R I Med J* 1979; **62:** 245.

30. Marwick C. Many physicians following own advice about not smoking. *JAMA* 1984; **252:** 2804.

31. Buechner JS, Perry DK, Scott HD, Freedman BE, Tierney JT, Waters WJ. Cigarette smoking behavior among Rhode Island physicians, 1963–83. *Am J Public Health* 1986; **76:** 285–86.

32. Burgess AM, Jr., Casey DB, Tierney JT. Cigarette smoking by Rhode Island physicians, 1963–1973: comparison with lawyers and other adult males. *Am J Public Health* 1978; **68:** 63–65.

33. Burgess AM, Jr., Casey DV, Tierney JT, DePalo P. Cigarette smoking by Rhode Island physicians: a fifteen year update. Percentage of physicians who smoke continues to decrease. *R I Med J* 1980; **63:** 345–47.

34. Burgess AM, Jr., Tierney JT. Rhode Island physicians' smoking habits revisited 1963–1968. *R I Med J* 1969; **52:** 437–40.

35. Burgess AM, Jr., Tierney JT. Bias due to nonresponse in a mail survey of Rhode Island physicians' smoking habits – 1968. *N Engl J Med* 1970; **282:** 908.

36. Murphy TH, Tierney JT. Current Status of Cigarette Smoking among Rhode Island Physicians. *R I Med J* 1963; **46:** 655–57.

37. Smith DR, Leggat PA. An international review of tobacco smoking in the medical profession: 1974–2004. *BMC Public Health* 2007; **7:** 115.

38. Greenwald P, Nelson D, Greene D. Smoking habits of physicians and their wives. *N Y State J Med* 1971; **71:** 2096–98.

39. The smoking study. A report of the attitudes and habits of California physicians with respect to cigarette smoking. *Calif Med* 1968; **109:** 339–44.

40. Wells KB, Lewis CE, Leake B, Ware JE, Jr. Do physicians preach what they practice? A study of physicians' health habits and counseling practices. *JAMA* 1984; **252:** 2846–48.

41. Fortmann SP, Sallis JF, Magnus PM, Farquhar JW. Attitudes and practices of physicians regarding hypertension and smoking: The Stanford Five City Project. *Prev Med* 1985; **14:** 70–80.

42. Linn LS, Yager J, Cope D, Leake B. Health habits and coping behaviors among practicing physicians. *West J Med* 1986; **144:** 484–89.

43. Thomas N. Smoking attitudes of New Haven county physicians: a survey. *Conn Med* 1968; **32:** 902–05.

44. Levitt EE, DeWitt KN. A survey of smoking behavior and attitudes of Indiana physicians. *J Indiana State Med Assoc* 1970; **63:** 336–39.

45. Snegireff LS, Lombard OM. Survey of smoking habits of Massachusetts physicians. *N Engl J Med* 1954; **250:** 1042–45.

46. Snegireff LS, Lombard OM. Smoking habits of Massachusetts physicians; five-year follow-up study (1954–1959). *N Engl J Med* 1959; **261:** 603–04.

47. Monson RR. Cigarette smoking by Massachusetts physicians – 1968. *N Engl J Med* 1970; **282:** 906–08.

48. Wyshak G, Lamb GA, Lawrence RS, Curran WJ. A profile of the health-promoting behaviors of physicians and lawyers. *N Engl J Med* 1980; **303:** 104–07.

49. Browning RH, Thorp D. Cigarettes. The Ohio Thoracic Society reports. *Ohio State Med J* 1969; **65:** 245–47.

50. Meighan SS, Weitman M. Smoking: habits and beliefs of Oregon physicians. *J Natl Cancer Inst* 1965; **35:** 893–98.

51. Weitman M, Meighan SS. Smoking patterns and specialty training of Oregon physicians. *Cancer* 1967; **20:** 974–82.

52. Boucot KR, Mausner JS. Smoking among the members of the Philadelphia County Medical Society. *Phila Med* 1964; **59:** 711–12.

53. Enstrom JE, Kanim LE. Smoking cessation among California physicians: an example of cancer control. *Prog Clin Biol Res* 1984; **156:** 255–64.

54. Lipp MR, Benson SG. Physician use of marijuana, alcohol, and tobacco. *Am J Psychiatry* 1972; **129:** 612–16.

55. Covey LS, Wynder EL. Smoking habits and occupational status. *J Occup Med* 1981; **23:** 537–42.

56. The impact of providing physicians with quit-smoking materials for smoking patients. *CA Cancer J Clin* 1981; **31:** 75–78.

57. National Clearinghouse for Smoking and Health: Survey conducted by the National Opinion Research Center Washington: US Public Health Service, 1968.

58. Bruce DL, Eide KA, Smith NJ, Seltzer F, Dykes MH. Characteristics of the American Society of Anesthesiologists' membership, 1967–1971. *Anesthesiology* 1974; **41:** 67–70.

59. Sterling TD, Weinkam JJ. Smoking characteristics by type of employment. *J Occup Med* 1976; **18:** 743–54.

60. Current trends: Smoking behavior and attitudes of physicians, dentists, nurses, and pharmacists, 1975. *MMWR Morb Mortal Wkly Rep* 1977; **26:** 185.

61. Survey of physicians' attitudes and practices in early cancer detection. *CA Cancer J Clin* 1985; **35:** 197–213.

62. Stellman SD, Boffetta P, Garfinkel L. Smoking habits of 800,000 American men and women in relation to their occupations. *Am J Ind Med* 1988; **13:** 43–58.

63. Brackbill R, Frazier T, Shilling S. Smoking characteristics of US workers, 1978–1980. *Am J Ind Med* 1988; **13:** 5–41.

64. Nelson DE, Giovino GA, Emont SL, Brackbill R, Cameron LL, Peddicord J, Mowery PD. Trends in cigarette smoking among US physicians and nurses. *JAMA* 1994; **271:** 1273–75.

65. Doctor, When did you have your last cigarette? *Med Tribune* 1965; **6:** 21.

66. 1966 survey results: Fewer doctors now smoke; patients often ignore advice. *Mod Med* 1966; **34:** 8, 14.

67. Special survey – How doctors take care of themselves. *Patient Care* 1976; **10:** 49–59.

68. McIlreath FJ, Cohen BM. Ventilatory performance of American physicians. *Am J Med Sci* 1966; **252:** 1–8.

69. Westling-Wikstrand H, Monk MA, Thomas CB. Some characteristics related to the career status of women physicians. *Johns Hopkins Med J* 1970; **127:** 273–86.

## Chapter 6

1. Rahman M, Fukui T. Biomedical publication – global profile and trend. *Public Health* 2003; **117:** 274–80.

2. Booth K, Faulkner A. Links between nurses and cigarette smoking? *Nurse Educ Today* 1986; **6:** 176–82.

3. Burgess AM, Jr., Tierney JT. Bias due to nonresponse in a mail survey of Rhode Island physicians' smoking habits – 1968. *N Engl J Med* 1970; **282:** 908.

4. Morra ME, Knobf MK. Comparison of nurses' smoking habits: the 1975 DHEW survey and Connecticut nurses, 1981. *Public Health Rep* 1983; **98:** 553–57.

5. Ohida T, Takemura S, Nozaki N, Kawahara K, Minowa M, Mochizuki Y. The validity of repeated mail surveys concerning smoking habits for Japanese physicians. *Nippon Koshu Eisei Zasshi* 2001; **48:** 573–83 [in Japanese].

6. Rodrigues GA, Galvao V, Viegas CA. Prevalence of smoking among dentists in the Federal District of Brasilia, Brazil. *J Bras Pneumol* 2008; **34:** 288–93.

7. Burgan SZ. Smoking behavior and views of Jordanian dentists: A pilot survey. *Oral Surg Oral Med Oral Pathol Oral Radiol Endod* 2003; **95:** 163–68.

8. Lodi G, Bez C, Rimondini L, Zuppiroli A, Sardella A, Carrassi A. Attitude towards smoking and oral cancer prevention among northern Italian dentists. *Oral Oncol* 1997; **33:** 100–04.

9. Boyle P. Tobacco smoking and the British doctors' cohort. *Br J Cancer* 2005; **92:** 419–20.

10. Clever LH, Arsham GM. Physicians' own health – some advice for the advisors. *West J Med* 1984; **141:** 846–54.

11. Yaacob I, Abdullah ZA. Smoking habits and attitudes among doctors in a Malaysian hospital. *Southeast Asian J Trop Med Public Health* 1993; **24:** 28–31.

12. Mausner JS. Smoking in medical students. A survey of attitudes, information, and smoking habits. *Arch Environ Health* 1966; **13:** 51–60.

13. Thomas CB, Ross DC, Higinbothom CQ. Precursors of hypertension and coronary disease among healthy medical students: discriminant function analysis. I. Using smoking habits as the criterion. *Bull Johns Hopkins Hosp* 1964; **115:** 174–94.

14. Smith DR, Leggat PA. An international review of tobacco smoking among medical students. *J Postgrad Med* 2007; **53:** 55–62.

15. Smith DR, Leggat PA. An international review of tobacco smoking among dental students in 19 countries. *Int Dent J* 2007; **57:** 452–58.

16. Elkind AK. Do nurses smoke because of stress? *J Adv Nurs* 1988; **13:** 733–45.

17. Rowe K, Clark JM. Evaluating the effectiveness of a smoking cessation intervention designed for nurses. *Int J Nurs Stud* 1999; **36:** 301–11.

18. Hope A, Kelleher CC, O'Connor M. Lifestyle practices and the health promoting environment of hospital nurses. *J Adv Nurs* 1998; **28:** 438–47.

19. Strobl J, Latter S. Qualified nurse smokers' attitudes towards a hospital smoking ban and its influence on their smoking behaviour. *J Adv Nurs* 1998; **27:** 179–88.

20. Brown MH, Kiss ME. Evaluation of competition as a method to recruit nurses into an employee self-help quit-smoking program. A failed experiment. *Cancer Nurs* 1987; **10:** 227–30.

21. World Health Organization website. *Tobacco Free Initiative (TFI)*. Available online at: www.who.int/tobacco/en/ (Accessed: 21 July 2010)

22. World Health Organization website. *What in the World Works? International Consultation on Tobacco and Youth, Final Conference Report*. Available online at: whqlibdoc.who.int/hq/2000/WHO_NMH_TFI_00.1.pdf (Accessed: 21 July 2010)

23. McCartan BE, Shanley DB. Policies and practices of European dental schools in relation to smoking; a ten-year follow-up. *Br Dent J* 2005; **198:** 423–25.

24. Stacey F, Heasman PA, Heasman L, Hepburn S, McCracken GI, Preshaw PM. Smoking cessation as a dental intervention: views of the profession. *Br Dent J* 2006; **201:** 109–13; discussion 99.

## Appendices

1. Schenker MB, Samuels SJ, Green RS, Wiggins P. Adverse reproductive outcomes among female veterinarians. *Am J Epidemiol* 1990; **132:** 96–106.

2. Tielen MJ, Elbers AR, Snijdelaar M, van Gulick PJ, Preller L, Blaauw PJ. Prevalence of self-reported respiratory disease symptoms among veterinarians in the Southern Netherlands. *Am J Ind Med* 1996; **29:** 201–07.

3. Gabel CL, Gerberich SG. Risk factors for injury among veterinarians. *Epidemiology* 2002; **13:** 80–86.

4. Susitaival P, Kirk JH, Schenker MB. Atopic symptoms among California veterinarians. *Am J Ind Med* 2003; **44:** 166–71.

5. Andersen CI, Von Essen SG, Smith LM, Spencer J, Jolie R, Donham KJ. Respiratory symptoms and airway obstruction in swine veterinarians: a persistent problem. *Am J Ind Med* 2004; **46:** 386–92.

6. Wilkins MJ, Bartlett PC, Judge LJ, Erskine RJ, Boulton ML, Kaneene JB. Veterinarian injuries associated with bovine TB testing livestock in Michigan, 2001. *Prev Vet Med* 2009; **89:** 185–90.

7. Harling M, Strehmel P, Schablon A, Nienhaus A. Psychosocial stress, demoralization and the consumption of tobacco, alcohol and medical drugs by veterinarians. *J Occup Med Toxicol* 2009; **4:** 4.

8. Fritschi L, Day L, Shirangi A, Robertson I, Lucas M, Vizard A. Injury in Australian veterinarians. *Occup Med (Lond)* 2006; **56:** 199–203.

9. Shirangi A, Fritschi L, Holman CD. Prevalence of occupational exposures and protective practices in Australian female veterinarians. *Aust Vet J* 2007; **85:** 32–38.

10. Smith DR, Leggat PA. Tobacco smoking by occupation in Australia: results from the 2004 to 2005 National Health Survey. *J Occup Environ Med* 2007; **49:** 437–45.

11. Smith DR, Leggat PA, Speare R. The latest endangered species in Australia: a tobacco-smoking veterinarian. *Aust Vet J* 2010; **88:** 369–70.

12. Poole JA, LeVan TD, Slager RE, Qiu F, Severa L, Yelinek J, *et al.* Bronchodilator responsiveness in swine veterinarians. *J Agromedicine* 2007; **12:** 49–54.

13. Webb E, Ashton H, Kelly P, Kamali F. Patterns of alcohol consumption, smoking and illicit drug use in British university students: interfaculty comparisons. *Drug Alcohol Depend* 1997; **47:** 145–53.

14. Hofmeister EH, Muilenburg JL, Kogan L, Elrod SM. Over-the-counter stimulant, depressant, and nootropic use by veterinary students. *J Vet Med Educ* 2010; **37:** 403–16.

# Index

www.ingramcontent.com/pod-product-compliance
Lightning Source LLC
Chambersburg PA
CBHW081417250726
48654CB00013B/1733